GOOD ~~~~ ~~~
COME FROM BAD TIMES

John Bruce (signature)

My Three Belly Button's

My Three Belly Button's

A true story of Cancer and Me,
By John Bruce

An open conversation of my battle with Cancer, the treatments, the recoveries, and the constant life challenges after diagnosis that changed my life forever. I hope I can provide some helpful insight to all those affected by Cancer and those that love them.

My Three Belly Button's
Cancer and Me

The cover picture is one of a Limber Pine in the north end of the Porcupine Hills that a friend sent to me with the following note.

"It is a lone tree growing out of a rock out crop with grass land all around it. As you can see it is weathered and broken and yet it survives (how, I don't know). I saw the tree a few months ago and thought of you ..."

I am weathered and broken yet I survive, but I am not alone in my journey, I have had much help along the way.

I have three beautiful children, a loving sister, mom and dad, and many great friends. My girlfriend of the past year and a half has been there for me any time I needed her. I am a Wildfire Prevention Officer/Fire Behaviour Specialist in Fort McMurray, Alberta. It is an honourable profession which I am grateful to have enjoyed these past twenty years. My co-workers have watched me fight this fire for the past four years. They have stood by me helplessly, watching and ready to offer assistance at any turn in the road. This is my story.

Dedications

I dedicate this book to Jeanette Lingley, without her strength and support the writing of this would not have been possible.

I thank my children, Caleb, Carly and David for giving me a reason to go on when I started to think there wasn't a reason left. I am so proud of the people you are, and will become.

I thank my Mom, Dad and Sister for being there day in day out when I needed them most.

For Russell, Barb, Colin and Oliver who have passed on due to Cancer since the beginning of my journey, you will be missed and I think of you often.

Table of Contents

Chapter 1

A Lump on My Throat

I am a survivor and this is my story so far. I am writing this for those that come after me, or those that have a loved one experiencing what I do not wish on my worst enemy. I am writing to see if this will help ease the pain and frustration in any way possible, both mine and yours. It is sort of a physical and emotional chronology of my battle with Cancer and the following battle with life to date. I must apologize ahead of time to those that were with me at the various stages of this story and may know the true account better then I. It is hard to remember at times and some events blend into others in the jumbled mess that is what remains of my chemo brained mind. I must admit I do have my faculties all about me, but that said, some pieces of the puzzle have been lost or misplaced and others substituted into a memory which has blurred in some areas. One day four summers ago I started to notice a swelling on my throat. I wrote it off as swollen glands at first. As time passed it grew slowly. When you see it every day you tend not to notice that it is indeed growing. Or you do notice it, but find yourself making excuses in a sort of blind denial of it all. With me, a close friend at work just blurted it out one day. She said that swelling on your neck is very noticeable, it is growing and you have to get it checked out by a Doctor now, not later. I promised that I would, took her advice and concern seriously, and finally stopped denying the possible problem and set up an appointment.

The doctor was very good and honest with me. He told me it might be nothing to worry about but the worst case scenario was that it may be Cancerous. He wanted me to see a specialist and they would take a sample of the growth and confirm either way. Still in denial, and hoping for the best but deep down sensing the worst, I waited anxiously for my appointment with the specialist in Edmonton. A couple of weeks later I was starting the beginning of my long journey to today.

The couple of weeks wait were spent on a rollercoaster of emotion. Is it nothing I thought, oh yes of course it's nothing, will I die I thought, what will I do? This was one of the hardest times in the whole cycle of ups and downs. Fear of the unknown. How much time do I have? I miss my kids. I am not ready to die yet. Maybe everyone will be better off if I die. What will I tell them? How will I tell them? Will it take long? Will it drag on? Maybe it's nothing and I am worrying for no reason. I am just being an idiot, working myself up over this. Who will show up at my funeral service? Will it be empty? Will it be full? What will they say? What will they think of me? I wish time would speed up. How much time do I have? Will I see my kids graduate? I should have never moved away from them. Maybe if I die quick it won't hurt as much. No, I can't die. I want to see them graduate and get married, I want to spoil their kids, I want, I want, I am losing it. Suck it up, it is out of your control, you will find out soon enough and make plans from there.

I was not very productive at work. It was good to keep busy, but hard to focus for any prolonged length of time. The first battle had begun and I was losing it. Finally the big day had arrived, and I was off to see the Specialist. A nervous tension filled me as I drove down the long highway thinking of what might be. It was almost a relief to register my arrival to see the Doctor at the hospital. I had been holding everything in at home, keeping my feelings hidden, pretending all was well, withdrawing to my room to be alone with my fears whenever I could.

That first Doctor was friendly enough but the whole meeting was a blur. He looked into my throat and seeing the telltale signs, he wasted no time. Pulling a needle out, he slid it into the lump on right side of my neck and withdrew a core type sample. He told me the results may take a little time to come from the lab and that if they came back positive for Cancer he would call me and would then be referring me to a Head and Neck Specialist if necessary.

Time passed slowly, waiting is not easy. This is a time where I couldn't be busy enough to keep my imagination from blowing up the worst possible scenarios in my head. You can only keep on going about your regular business as you would any other day. It's not the type of conversation you have at coffee time or around the water cooler. Cancer has always held a type of taboo associated with it and is not something the average crowd wants to discuss or chat about. Most of the people I worked with were quite young and just starting their lives with no thoughts of something so dark as to tear away their sense of immortality. I felt very alone and helpless. The "what ifs" kept pulling me down. It is hard enough to get through on your own. Rather than bringing my burden to those I loved and having them deal with the pain and uncertainty. I kept the information to a small few at work, who had seen the growth and were aware I was getting it checked out.

Chapter 2

Diagnosis

Hours became days, and then the phone call came. In some ways it was welcome, knowing this was finally it, as the wait was excruciatingly painful, both mentally stressing and emotionally taxing. In other ways it was like awaiting a death sentence, for the floor to drop and the noose to tighten. I said hello and waited silently. There was no small talk just a direct business like voice stating the facts, I have Squamous Cell Carcinoma which is a variety of skin Cancer and my file has been forwarded to Dr. Williams who is a specialist in the field of surgeries related to head and neck cancers. I will be receiving an appointment shortly for an assessment and maybe further sampling of the tumor.

You can imagine this is a bit hard to take. It is a good thing that I found out the news when I had gone back to my hotel room during lunch from a course I was attending in Edmonton. Being alone at the time allowed me some time to let my emotions go freely and get some of them out.

I just sort of stood there, dead phone in hand staring at the wall feeling trapped, helpless and defeated. All the bad thoughts came rushing back from the weeks previous. The nightmare was not a dream, it was real now. I was at a loss as to what to do next so I just stood there alternating from crying, feeling sorry for myself, feeling pain and anguish, becoming enraged with the possibility I wouldn't see my kids graduate. Then denial as to the seriousness of what I just heard, not believing that anything would change, wondering about my own mortality.

The two hardest thoughts I had, were related to how I was going to tell my parents and my children. I can remember the phone conversation with my Mom; it was one I will never forget. I just sort of said hi and then blurted it out, "I have Cancer". Didn't know what to do or say after that, we just sort of broke down, regained composure, than broke down again. Standing there fighting to keep our composure but sliding into crying and worry of what might be, I finally had to say goodbye and hang up before I had a total meltdown.

Now I really felt lost, I needed something solid to keep my mind occupied as an active imagination with news like this just seems to run out of control and make things ten times as bad as they perhaps are. The phone rang again and I answered. It was a friend of mine, a work mate that was attending the course with me. I had told him I had been expecting some news and he was worried for me so had decided to call as I was absent from the afternoons session of the course. I told him I would arrive shortly, that I was just held up. I tried to block the reality out of my head and returned to the course. Although I think it helped for a little while, my mind kept drifting back to the Cancer. At break I informed my friends what I had found out and went to talk to the instructor. I told her that I apologize in advance if I leave the class in the middle of a session, but I had just received some very bad news and I don't know if I could continue with the course.

I lasted a while, but soon left as I couldn't keep the fearful thoughts out of my head of my world ending. The idea of breaking down and crying amongst my peers was not one I wanted to act on at this time so I whispered goodbye and left. My friend said he would call me after class and check in with me. I went back to the hotel room. Stretched out on the bed and put a pillow over my eyes with which to block out the world. I wanted sleep to take me so I could escape. This turned out to be wishful thinking. It felt impossible to turn my mind off, negative thoughts rushed through me. I think I finally gave in and sat up. I turned on the TV. I watched but did not take anything in. I was completely occupied with the events of the afternoon and feeling sorry for myself, poor me. I still had to tell my kids. I can't remember how this happened, I think I called their mother and told her, and then she relayed the bad news on to them. Having being separated from her for a few years I really appreciated this gesture. It is such a sad thought. I have wiped it from my mind. I wish it on no one. Funny as I sit here writing about it I still can't put into words or even imagine how to go about telling your own kids that you have Cancer. I am at a complete and utter loss to it.

I don't think any of it really sunk in. The whole experience has a surreal flavor to it. It all becomes a bit of a dream, one long bad dream. That night I went out to escape. I went out for a great steak dinner and drink at a high end downtown restaurant with a few close friends. Good food, good wine, good company, topped off by a dessert nip of 12 year old single malt scotch to finish. For the most part the conversation stayed away from my issues but occasionally it would rear its ugly head and dominate for a while. Funny how that is, it has been almost four years now and it is hard to make it through a night with old friends now, without it coming up in conversation at least once in an evening. I guess I may as well get used to that monkey never leaving my back, and look at it from the perspective that at least people are talking about it now and it's not treated like the taboo plague of the past that it seemed to be, all hush hush and talked about in whispers.

The next day I could say I had a nice evening, but now the fun was over and it was time to get serious about this. It was time to inform people, such as my boss, my friend the admin lady who told me to get checked out, some of my closest friends and my family Doctor who started me on this journey.

My boss told me to go on sick leave; I told him I would like to continue working while I am waiting to find out what will happen next in order to keep my mind occupied. I continued to go to the course another day or so but could not finish it. Between the mass of emotions I felt and the phone ringing off and on with caring friends and/or a list of new appointments to go to, I had to leave.

Chapter 3

A Little Getaway

After seeing the new Specialist, it was determined that further investigation would be required into seeing how far the Cancer had spread. Multiple biopsies were required from my throat, mouth and nasal areas. This made sense to me and I didn't really think much of it. I figured if they were going to fix the problem it made sense that they determine the extent of what they were dealing with so I was right bought in with the program. During this time my ex and I thought it would be a good time to take the kids on a trip somewhere to have some fun before the hard stuff started. I remembered the first biopsy taken by needle from my neck so I was very happy when I found out that they would be knocking me out for this one. As I lay on the table just about ready for the anesthetic, I asked my doctor if I could go to Mexico before treatment, to which he responded yes as I fell into unconsciousness. I awoke from the procedure feeling fine and none the worse for wear looking forward to telling my kids that they were getting to miss a week of school because we were going to Mexico the following week.

The trip was a good one, sunshine and relaxation being with my children. The whole idea of Cancer and the stress it provides you is a bit fatiguing. At times I just wanted to sit and watch my children or nothing in particular for a while. Just float away with my thoughts to nowhere in particular enjoying the moment. I would recommend this type of trip to anyone. It doesn't have to be to anywhere exotic but it must give you the opportunity to pamper and spoil yourself one last time because the trip ahead is going to be rough. It is not going to be joyful. It is at times going to be painful, both physically and mentally. This is not something you just take an aspirin for and walk away feeling all better from, this is Cancer with a capital "C".

Chapter 4

The Tumor

I have had excellent health care providers from many different hospitals and many different areas of profession over the last few years and the best thing I can say regarding them is that the information they presented me was never sugar coated. It was always timely and straight up, describing clearly to me the challenge I was about to face. For many of you and your loved ones, this will be the hardest thing you have ever gone through or will ever go through again in your life. Survival is not a guarantee but you will have the best chance at it, and it can be accomplished, if you stay positive and do the work that is asked of you. Sometimes you may feel there is no hope and this is when good loving support from those close to you will lift you up and carry your burden for a while. Let them help you, show them or ask them when you need help. It is not a sign of weakness to show frailty but rather a show of strength.

Now the tumor on my neck to begin this story was a small lump maybe 3 cm long by 1.5 cm wide, slightly raised and located on the right side of my throat where it meets the jaw in an area most of us may find swollen glands when we are sick with a cold or flu. It was raised up at most a centimeter so it blended in very well and was not noticeable to many. Once it had reached this visible size it started to grow quite fast. After the surgical biopsies I was supposed to have an appointment to have baseline testing done and get pictures of my mouth area as well as test my ability to talk and swallow. I was also supposed to have another appointment with my surgeon specialist and get some assessments and such at the Cross Cancer Institute in Edmonton. Many people on my new team were getting ready to help me.

One problem was encountered during this time. My tumor had decided it would not wait and began to grow at an uncontrollable rate to the point where it started to cause me excruciating pain. Once it reached a size of approximately 15 x 20 cm and swelled up about 4 cm running from my tonsils tucked up under my chin along my throat, to now my right ear lobe it began to cause pain. Until this time it was hard to look at in the mirror, but the physical pain was not there.

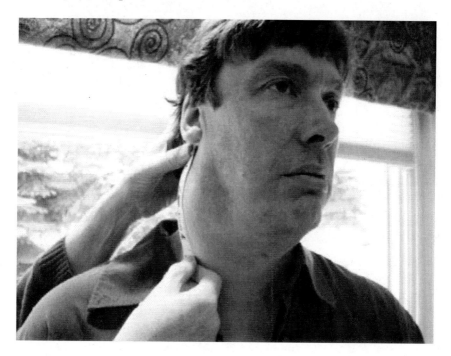

Chapter 5

Time for the Emergency Ward

I had a jar of Tylenol 3 with codeine that my Doctor prescribed for me if I started to experience pain and I started to eat them like candy. At my worst I took nineteen tablets of Tylenol 3, and it did nothing but take a slight edge off the pain. I had been staying at my parents in the city to be near the Doctor in case it started to get out of hand. My specialist appointment was approaching the following week but not soon enough for the Cancer and the pain it created. They took me to their doctor to see what he could do for me and he prescribed morphine pills to help alleviate what I was feeling to no avail. It just got worse and worse except now I was becoming incoherent with the medication and babbling nonsense, harder by the moment for my parents to deal with. All I had to do was make it a couple more days to my specialist appointment but it was too much. Too much to handle, my parents took me to the emergency at the hospital my Doctor worked out of. There I remember the ER nurse asking me "on a scale of one to ten how much pain are you having" and my reply being 8 or 9, then she gave me a nice big shot of happiness in the form of a loaded syringe full of morphine that made all the misery go away, if only for a short time.

That was near the beginning of December and would be the last time I ventured out from behind those walls for the next couple of months. I am not sure how long my stay in Emergency was, I only remember fragments of this time. It was peaceful and the pain was kept at bay. I would drift in and out of consciousness in a dreamlike state. I remember a guy complaining behind the curtain next to me that he had been at a crack and meth party all weekend and that he was complaining of heavy abdominal pain, the nurse asked him the question "On a scale of one to ten how would you rate the pain" his answer was a whiny "ten" and I still had the ability to have a red neck thought to myself, give him a placebo and bring me some more morphine. Cold thought yes, maybe, but I had endured such pain over the past few days that I wanted to take out my anger on someone or something. Again the nurse returned and I may or may not have voiced my thoughts filled with delirium but I laughed at the thought and drifted off to her reassuring comforting voice until the next needle.

My pain stabilized for how long I do not know. I was moved to a room in the wards in preparation and wait for surgery. The rooms were full so they stuffed three beds into the room I occupied with my closest neighbor having similar issues to mine except that his tumor was on his voice box. His name was Russell and he would join me at many junctures in the future of our treatments.

The team I initially expected to see was no longer an option as the Cancer had taken a strong hold and was at Stage 3 aggressively growing faster by the day. The only option left was immediate surgery. Then too follow it up with radiation and chemotherapy, foregoing the standard baseline and info session appointments. Up the ladder of priority I climbed. I guess it's nice to have some clout when you are waiting in a line up for dinner at a fancy restaurant, but when you are in line for radical surgery of the head and throat it doesn't have the same appeal. Oh well, they had me on a solid diet of morphine so things were quite relaxed for me at this time. I would probably say my support system of those people I loved had more issues at this time then I. I say this because I wasn't capable of truly grasping the seriousness of the situation regarding what I was about to endure. It all just sounded like the logical, matter of fact, path to go down. The complexity of it all broke down into simple logic, my emotions dulled by the morphine.

Chapter 6

The Surgery

In preparation for the surgery my father and I spent some time with a lady from the speech and swallow team at the hospital. Together we looked at diagrams depicting what was going to be done to me. Looking back on it now I think this must have been torture for my Dad but for me the conversation seemed matter of fact and it all made good sense. I was numb to the seriousness of what was about to take place, and I am thankful for that. It went sort of like this in my mind;

First, they will make an incision in your neck below your right ear and slit round your throat below your Adams apple and then up again to about an inch below your left ear.

Second, they will make another incision from this first incision below your Adams apple straight up to your mouth splitting your lower lip in two.

Third, they will open the flaps up that are now formed, pull a tooth in your lower jaw then break it in line with the vertical incision so that they may spread your mouth open and access the tumor in your throat.

Fourth, they will cut out the cancerous tumor, but this will leave a hole or cavity in the back of your throat that needs to be filled.

Fifth, they will take a large graft about the size of 1/3 of a deck of playing cards from the inside of your lower arm to fill this hole. You only need one major artery and vein in your arm, and you have two there, so they will remove one set to maintain a blood supply to the graft.

Sixth, they will harvest a skin graft from your quad, harvesting skin cells with something like a cheese grater, and use this to cover the graft area on your arm.

Ok, so how long will it take for the whole surgery I asked? About eight to ten hours was the reply. Now this seems like a long time to be in surgery. I agree it is, but, my mentality was that sounds about right so let's do it. The whole thing just seemed so routine to me. I had no clue of what was to come. Had I known what was coming in the next couple of days I would have asked for a last meal so to speak. A meal consisting of some steak like object, that I could chew nice and long savoring every morsel, and then lick the plate after.

What occurred was a surgery with complications that lasted not 8 to 10 hours but rather 17 hours of pure miracles. Looking back I don't know how I survived. It also turns out that I have an irregular heartbeat which they happened across during this procedure just to add one more problem to the situation. This time is very blurry for me indeed floating in and out of consciousness in ICU and then in my new ward for recovery. I finally had some realization of what this was all about and it became all too clear to me at that moment.

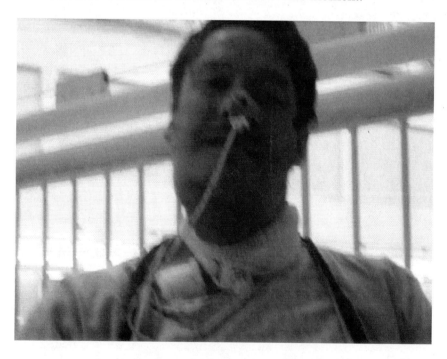

I was in a room, nurses and doctors floated in and out checking this, looking at that, sticking a needle in there. I just laid there shaking the cobwebs off. My youngest son, age 12, didn't recognize me very well due to the swelling. That said, he commented at a later date that he was expecting that I would have looked a lot worse. So there I sat propped up in bed. Let's go through the new attachments I was given. I had a feeding tube in my nose hooked up to the IV station, I had 3 or 4 lymph node drains attached to my neck area to drain the fluid built up from the surgery, my right upper chest had a couple of wires or something sticking out where they could check the veinal and arterial rhythms of the graft inserted in my throat, I had a trache inserted below my Adams apple to ensure my airway was not compromised. Now that brings back a memory of how that trache was installed. Just before I went under for surgery the trache was installed. I remember being told something to the effect that it had to be inserted prior to me becoming unconscious in case my throat collapsed and the airway was blocked. Again, I am not positive on the reasoning, but airways are important and I will leave it at that. All I remember is that it was a very uncomfortable thing having someone cut into your esophagus when you are completely aware of it. I seem to remember holding my breath as he cut in. As soon as the trache was in, anesthetic was released and I was out. Back to the list we continue. I had a protective removable cast type item which was very strong and form fitting on my left arm to protect the area of the main graft, and my left quad graft area was bandaged on my leg. I was held together by a plate in my chin and staples and stiches around my neck and from my wrist to elbow. Pretty impressive scars I might add. IVs and tubes and wires were coming out of everywhere.

Chapter 7

The First Few Days

Pain, I would give it a ten out of ten, morphine or no morphine, it was excruciating. As if the physical pain and shock to my body wasn't enough, I had the roommate from hell. A miserable old so and so that had I had a gun handy no one would have said a word if he went on his merry way to the other side. Your first couple days are crucial to survival and the way things were going he was driving me and the nurses of the ward insane and over the edge at every opportunity. I literally pleaded with the nurses to move me. I couldn't talk so I wrote notes pleading with them that if they didn't move me soon I didn't know if I had the strength to make it. He played his radio 24/7 and soiled himself and the bed as often as possible just to create misery for those employed in helping him. Please for your sake and the sake of others in there with you. Please show patience and be a good patient no matter what happens it can only benefit you in the long run.

After a couple of days in hell I was spared and moved to another room with an older gentleman who was very quiet and easy going and now my recovery could begin. Pain, pain and more pain. Still swollen and having a constant pounding headache thanks to my "best friend" in the other room. I had for some reason or other decided that maybe it was the morphine giving me the headaches so I tried to avoid it. I had been moved from having the self- administered dose where you click the little button and if it has been long enough since your last shot it will give you another one. I remember sitting there for just about all my waking moments holding onto that thing and clicking away hoping that the shot had reloaded and I could float away once more if only for just a little while. Then to having the irrational thought in my head that all my headaches were due to taking it. I started to hold off on the shot as long as I could take it and then it would have little effect and I would lie there head pounding in misery. A nurse took a few moments to explain possible reasons why I was having problems and why the pain medications seemed to be having little effect. She explained that it is much easier to combat the pain if you keep the medication levels at a constant timing and the dosage in a maintenance basis. Instead of letting the pain get too far out of hand, and beyond the control of a dose. This way you don't have to overcome the pain but rather just keep on top of it with each dose. Once I realized the sense of this, I went back to a regular dose and the pain became managed at a level I could deal with in short order. Once your body has healed to a certain level, these pain issues will alleviate, and then you can start cutting the doses and slowly wean yourself away from it.

Now I could truly start to think about recovery.

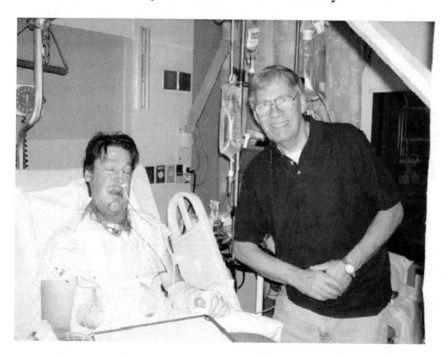

Christmas was approaching in a couple of weeks, and with it was an unrealistic hope of being at home for it. I mentioned earlier that there is work involved in getting better and this is where the support of all around you, health care workers, family and friends alike can all lend a hand to get you on your way and assist you wherever possible. From the moment I was showing any sign of capability to do anything towards my recovery, someone was there pushing me. This is a great thing because as like most of you, when you are extremely worn out and tired, and then given an opportunity to sit on the beach in the nice hot sun, or say play a busy game of Frisbee, most of you I assume would pick the stretched out lazily in the sun choice. The thing is that this type of mentality can do you more harm than good. On top of it all, the morphine is making you feel a bit lazy like, so it takes a good deal of prodding and probing to kick your butt off the bed. First was to get the legs going and body moving again. You need to get the circulation going again before pooling and clotting of blood occurs in your arteries from lack of movement. We don't need any nasty blood clots breaking loose and screwing up all the good work those Doctors just performed.

Chapter 8

Baby Steps

So in comes the little lady with the belt like leash thing that is attached to her around the waist, and soon to be wrapped around my waist, to get me on my feet and walking again. When or if I fall, she will catch me, is how the theory works. Now this took a bit for my mind to comprehend. I took physics in high school long ago and just couldn't see how this was going to work, other than badly, if I did fall. She was at most about 5'6" maybe 120 lbs. and I was 6'1" and 220 lbs plus. I felt okay with it though, as she had a confidence about her, and I figured she had done this before so I went along with it. Remember I still had a trache in my throat and could not speak at this moment, so there isn't going to be much warning if I went for a face plant. The experiment however, was a success. I think I made it about 20 or 30 meters before I ran out of energy, then took a rest leaning on my helper and then dragged myself back to bed exhausted until tomorrow. Little victory's is all I can say. Take any progress you can and look forward to a better day tomorrow.

Prior to surgery, I took some things related to our everyday life for granted, such as speech and swallowing. It is something so basic, that as a baby you instinctively started to shovel stuff into your mouth, eating everything and anything that you could wrap your little fingers around. Speech was a work in progress but it just sort of happens one day that you start to talk and some of us never knew when to shut up sticking our foot in our mouths from time to time. I awoke from surgery with these abilities gone. I had to learn them all over again. The anatomy of my mouth and throat was changed forever. Some muscles were removed outright, others were partially removed, some were severed, nerves were removed, and nerves were cut and so on.

Chapter 9

What Happened to Me

To give you an idea of the changes, I will describe them as I understand them to be today, in as simple terms as possible. The easiest way to start is to say prior to the surgery, I had a 15 and a half neck size. After the surgery I had a 13 and a half neck size with the two inch difference taken from the right side of my neck. I do mean taken, it was carved off the one side, all diseased tissue removed. There is a thing called the vocal fold in your throat which is made up of two flaps which vibrate together generating the sound which you know as your voice. During the surgery one of these flaps was paralyzed as the tumor had encroached upon it and had to be removed from that area. This left it so the flaps would not be able to vibrate against each other, which would result in me talking at most with a raspy whisper for a voice, if any at all. The doctors decided at that time to turn the still functional fold and move it closer to the other one so that it could vibrate against it with a hopeful result of my voice having a better chance of existence and possible normalcy. I am thinking this was one of the hiccups in surgery that stretched it out to 17 hours from the 8 to 10 hours in length initially predicted.

My jaw had to be vertically split in two, pulled apart and then realigned and joined back in place by a metal plate to ensure the bone had a chance to heal together. I would give them an A plus on this one, but the fact is, it is impossible to realign your teeth exactly how they were and this makes chewing interesting to say the least. Over the years your teeth wear together fitting upper and lower jaws together in a form fitting manner. You can imagine how difficult it would be to break and unhinge your lower jawbone and then put it back together perfectly so that each tooth aligns as it once was with the matching area on the upper row. Fitting perfectly together, like a hand sliding into a favorite baseball glove. This alone would be considered a miracle in itself, unrealistic as it is. The implication of this new bite is that sometimes two teeth hit each other with force, the alignment being slightly off where one wants to give way to the other. If you can imagine the feeling of your tooth almost snapping as they collide, and the pain and discomfort associated with that, you would agree that at times this can be a bit unsettling. Oh well life goes on, little troubles are just that, in the big scope of things. One thing you will learn fast in this world of Cancer and recovery is that it doesn't take long to look around and see someone worse off then you are.

The right side of my tongue was paralyzed and many of the nerves deadened not to return again. It just sort of drooped on the one side, they may have removed a little from the base of it in the back of my mouth, I am not completely sure. If I bit into it, sometimes I wouldn't notice until I saw the blood coming out the corners of my mouth. The right side SCM muscle along with a good portion of the scalene muscles and tonsils were also removed with the tumor of infected tissue. Many portions of the right side of my mouth inside and out had nerves damaged or removed.

A couple of weeks after surgery I started to get shocks out of nowhere occurring on my tongue and mouth area and was told the nerves must be growing back. It was as if someone had dragged their feet across the carpet and touched me on the face. You wouldn't believe how invaluable your tongue is in the process of swallowing and chewing. The tongues function is not only taste but as a muscle it moves the food around your mouth, without any real thinking on your part, and pushes the food to areas of your teeth that are most appropriate and efficient for chewing. After the food is ground to an appropriate consistency, it helps press the food to the roof of your mouth and pushes it back down to your throat where another group of muscles take over in synchronicity to make up what you know as your swallow.

Moving right along, and by the looks of the graft scar on my left forearm, I would say it must have been a good ¼ inch or 5 mm thick and a rectangle of about 7 cm long by 5 cm wide. One of the main arteries and vein pairs in the forearm was also removed with this to ensure blood flow was available for the graft. This scar is about a cm wide and goes up from my wrist to the inside of my elbow. The graft was then rolled up, much like a donut, and stuffed into the hole left by the tumor's removal. This practice was developed a few years before I arrived at the U of A Hospital, by some of the very same Doctors who were operating on me, so in this case I was lucky to be an Albertan in the presence of this improved technology and knowledge base. The vein and artery then had to be rejoined with the circulatory system in order to provide blood flow to the graft. This is done by slicing down your neck, from in my case just below the right ear, all the way down through the right trapezoid muscle and into your arterial network in the upper chest. Monitors were left in place to ensure the circulation was maintained because no blood flow means you have a dead graft or chunk of flesh in your throat which again can't be a good thing. During this exercise, my right vagus nerve was also severed along with many feelings on the entire right side of my neck and upper shoulder area. This nerve is critical to many bodily functions and one day I may fully understand the full effect of this occurrence, but not yet today.

Then there was the cheese grater graft on the upper quad of my left leg covering an area of approximately 10 cm by 15 cm. I say cheese grater, because that is basically what it is, they harvest skin cells from your leg leaving a raw scraped area behind which heals quite fast, but remains lightly visible for many years to come. It was the least intrusive of all my wounds and utilized to cover up the wound on my left arm allowing it to heal faster.

The trache deserves more mention. As I said, I was awake when they inserted it just prior to my surgery. It was cut into the area at the base of my throat just above my sternum. A hollow tube the size of your standard pen, yes just like in the MASH episode where Hawkeye does a trache insertion in the field it is really the same principle and a simple contraption that allows you to breathe. It all makes sense now looking in the mirror and wondering about how I looked with my jaw and throat all splayed open during surgery. I guess your airway would be a bit compromised, so to speak, without it. Some of the issues with a trache after the fact are a story in themselves and I will elaborate further as we move along in my recovery. I just wanted to paint a picture for you of what was done.

Chapter 10

Starting to Heal

Back to recovery, after accomplishing the great feat of travelling 20 to 30 meters under my own leg power it was on to bigger and better things. My progress in walking showed each day as I made it a little further each time finally graduating to being released off my leash and allowed to run free in the halls of the hospital. That said, it would still be a while yet before I had the strength and confidence combined, to venture beyond the security of the hospital ward. Completing a couple laps at a time of the ward sufficed for my exercise in the absence of my father coming to visit and taking me for a walk out in the hospital halls. Preparation for a walk was quite the event. Because of the cast on one arm protecting the graft, IVs on the other arm, nasal feeding tube, trache and such, I had to sort of drape a housecoat onto my shoulders and carefully secure it in place over my gown in order to be presentable in the public areas of the hospital. Seeing small children stare on occasion was something to think about, but understandable considering the swelling and stitches.

I mention the nasal tube in place, all the nutrients you could ask for in a bag dripped slowly into the back of your throat over the course of an hour. I was on a 3000 calorie diet of vanilla flavored liquid of life. I never could understand the vanilla flavoring as it never hit my taste buds unless I happened to burp it up, then it was just a disgusting reminder of what you were living on. I had a right to complain about something I figure, if only in the odd passing comment to my family and friends. That said, your body uses a lot of energy to rebuild itself after such trauma and I was shedding on average a pound per day in doing so. You could say my body was feeding on itself. It is a good thing that I had some extra pounds to lose, if I had been my goal weight I would have faded away to nothing before I got started on this exercise.

Most of my day was spent propped up in bed. I couldn't lie flat as it felt like I was going to choke on my own throat. It was a very strange feeling, as if someone had wrapped a hand around it and squeezed just enough to cause discomfort. Also, any liquid or saliva remnants in my throat made me gag and feel like I was going to drown so I had to spit it up. I would go through about three little Kleenex boxes a day. I had the bed and pillows set up so I was sitting pretty much straight up. Any head tilt backwards caused me to have a choking feeling and my head was too heavy to lift by my neck on its own without support.

Many different tests, x-rays, and such had me stretched out flat on my back uncomfortably on an examining table where I required assistance from whoever was there to put a hand under my neck to help lift my head off the table. It was like having an anchor attached to the back of your head. I would strain but didn't have the strength to lift it on my own.

Sleeping was very interesting, and challenging to say the least. Most days sleep would come from exhaustion. I slept sitting up. It reminded me of being back in school at a boring lecture where your head started to bob forward and sway, then it would flip back jerking you awake. Because I felt like drowning and choking if it tilted back at all, it was very hard to find an angle I could drift off in. Then since I was so vertical my head would fall forward with a similar result, sleep did not come easy. If it wasn't for medication I don't think I could have gotten more than an hour or so at a time, and that would be from passing out due to sheer exhaustion. The nurses were fantastic to me. They would chat to me quietly sometimes late into the night trying to take my mind off the misery and then the medication would start to kick in and off I would go, drifting into some faraway place, peaceful and quiet.

My life was now broken into four hour segments, as this was the frequency required for my medication. Some nights I would just drift off around 3AM, and in they would come with my dose of medication and I would stir and awaken. The nurses would do their best to come in quietly without disturbing me when I was sleeping. Most of the meds were administered through my IV in the night so they would quietly change the fluid and medication bags, reset everything and try to let me sleep through it whenever possible.

One of my least favorite things was the little IV administered bag of potassium, I think it was called. This always felt as if it was burning a new path in my veins each time I received it. My favorite time was when it was time for my shot of morphine, as this made me so relaxed and pain free in an almost euphoric manner. I can see how someone could become addicted to this feeling, and for a while I certainly felt that way. There are rules around such medications that nurses adhere to in a very strict manner and will not waiver from no matter how hard you whine or complain of the pain. I would get a couple of Tylenol with Codeine (T3) in between my shots of morphine which were given every four hours. As I said, this was my favorite time. The nurse could run her watch by me as I would be buzzing her the minute the clock turned to the next allowable dose. It was distracting when visitors were there and I would be clock watching. Now before you get all excited about this, you should recognize that the Tylenol barely took the edge off the pain and this was the only thing closely related to a happy pain free time I would have for months to come.

My daily routine included many needles. One in the stomach area I think was a blood thinner reducing the possibility of clots. Morphine every four hours in the bicep which after a while was completely bruised looking from elbow to shoulder. Blood work every couple days to test for hospital super bugs, kidney function and so on. Then there was the changing of the IV line every few days which became quite the challenge as veins started to shy away from the needles or completely disappear. I was basically a human pin cushion.

Chapter 11

My First Meal

Before my first meal after the surgery I was very apprehensive. There were so many things to remember in order to swallow without choking to death on whatever was put in front of me. There I was, cast on my lower left forearm and wrist, IV stuck in the right arm, Trache in swollen throat, lymph node drains hanging off me, stitches everywhere psyching myself up for the attempt. The meal arrived on a covered plate like you would find during room service at a hotel. The smell was fantastic. I was hungry and tired of the vanilla flavored nose drink which was my only sustenance of the past couple weeks. I lifted the lid in anticipation and almost cried. Sitting on the plate before me was a mound of mashed potatoes, hamburger steak and peas with gravy. I couldn't believe it, was this some sort of cruel joke I thought. There was no way in hell I could come close to swallowing what was before me. I would have been lucky to swallow a bit of cream soup and here was a meal. I was depressed and distraught. It was a mistake, these things happen, your health providers are human after all I thought to myself. Let it go, was all I could do. After talking to my speech and swallow therapist, we managed to get the meal changed to something I could attempt eating at last. I remember my mother being there when it arrived and my speech and swallow therapist, saying she would be up soon to see how I have done. In order to swallow I had to take in a breath and hold it, cover the hole on the trache, take one spoon of the food into my mouth on the left side, so that the unparallized side of my tongue could do its job without losing track of the food in my mouth and swallow hard. Sounds easy, doesn't it? Who would have thought so much work was involved in swallowing. Initially I struggled and choked, and when

I choked, I coughed, and liquid from the soup would squirt out from around my trache tube, soaking the wound and surrounding dressings. Not a very sanitary looking thing, but the wound could still be cleaned after the meal. I gave up. I was so frustrated with scooping a spoonful of soup just so I could choke and cough my brains out. Instead I asked my Mom to help and for the first time since I was a baby my mother fed me. I felt utterly helpless and embarrassed at the same time but I knew I had to eat and tomorrow would be another day to try for myself. Much to my prides disappointment, this wouldn't be the last time in my recovery that I would have to ask for a helping hand.

Determined I could do it on my own, I persisted and finally managed a clumsy semblance of something that looked sort of like eating. The faster I conquered eating and swallowing, the faster I would be able to get rid of the vanilla nose tube treats that I enjoyed so much, and this thought was a great incentive. This dream had to become reality faster than it should have, because one night in my sleep I pulled the tube out from my nose. Dreaming away my arm became caught up in it, and when I shifted in my sleep, I pulled it loose. My first thought upon waking and discovering this, was freedom, finally. Oh it felt good not to have that thing in my face. I wasn't thinking of the possible repercussions which became clear quickly when my speech and swallow therapist arrived that morning. She didn't look completely happy with this new development and asked me to explain what happened. I told her I had ripped it out in my sleep and she said it would be difficult to get a new one put in. I smiled on the inside until I learned the consequences of this action was that I was going to have to work harder on my swallow because now all my sustenance had to come from food and I still needed over 3000 calories a day to maintain recovery.

I have always loved food, but there were times when I didn't care if I saw another morsel.

Chapter 12

ECG Error Trauma Team Activation Panic Alert

When you are in a situation such as myself, stuck in the hospital after such a traumatic surgery people consider your situation very serious indeed. You may not really grasp such a concept as medication may be blurring the extent of what has just occurred. Now when I had surgery, it was discovered that my heart had an arrhythmia or an irregular beat. I am not sure if this was a pre-existing condition or if this was a result of the trauma my body had just gone through. Regardless of this fact, that is what the reality was and I would have to live with it. One day I lay in bed and a nurse came in with an ECG machine to take a script. She had never met me before and was unaware of my history. She was only aware that she was to take this script and report the findings. So we began.

Out came the stickers and wires. ECG machines come with a lot of stickers which are attached to wires. These will be stuck all over your body so that the machine can register your heart rate, type of rhythm, and such. Keep an eye on all the stickers as there are many and it is easy to miss one in the removal process which may become welded to your skin after a while if gone unnoticed. Anyway, back to the story of the ECG nurse. Unknown to her I guess I had a very irregular beat that day, which would be of no surprise to those who know me, because I have always marched to the beat of my own drum. Upon viewing my script, this set off the alarm bells in her and she proceeded to fly out the room and hit the alarm alert for the trauma team. All of a sudden there were announcements going over the hospital intercom for the trauma team on standby to activate and meet at room 3F which just so happened to be my number. The head floor nurse Peggy came rushing in and there I sat, stickers from head to toe calm and natural looking as could be considering the circumstance. This whole thing was a great surprise to her as she had seen me not 15 minutes earlier, and I was fine. She looked at me sitting there and asked if I felt ok, I said yes then she put two and two together and went out to stand down the team and explain to the ECG nurse my situation. That was enough excitement for ward 3.

Chapter 13

Rebuild and Weight Sustaining 184 in Drayton

I left the hospital on a mission, I had a couple of months to regain or sustain as much weight as possible and build my strength up as best as I could before it was time to continue my treatment with radiation and chemotherapy at the Cross Cancer Institute.

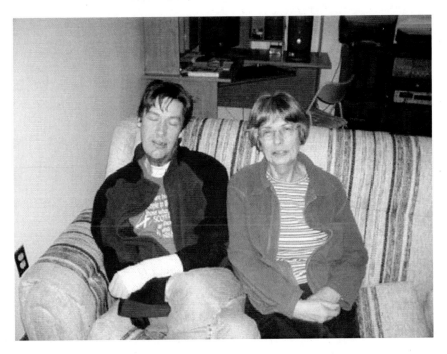

I had many challenges, the first being that I had to learn to swallow again.

I needed my 3000 calories. The anatomy of my throat had being changed during the surgery and localized paralysis in my mouth and tongue did not help matters. I had to mentally visualize how each bite of food would go down, and then follow the steps of a proper swallow. It is easy if you have been eating all your life and everything is in the right place for you, but that was not the case anymore. Some days I wanted to throw my food against the wall, slam my fists, and scream. This didn't matter though. The work still had to be done. Thank goodness for my 2500 calorie shake. It would take me an hour or two to drink down but left me with a manageable volume of calories to chew.

I went to physiotherapy and walked for exercise, slowly building my speed and stamina up to a point where I could motor around pretty good. I finally managed a pace, where I could complete a five kilometers walk in about 45 minutes on average. I was walking much like you would complete a slow jog. Every day I would walk further and faster. Sometimes my body would scream out, stop and sit for a while, and that is just what I would do. I had spots identified on my route that were perfect for vegetation breaks when needed. I went home at 184 lbs and headed out to the Cross cancer Institute at 184 pounds with some stamina and strength rebuilt and ready to fight another day. I knew the hard part was yet to come, the surgery was no cake walk but I needed to dig down and ready myself for the real battle.

Chapter 14

Introduction to the Cross

The Cross Cancer Clinic in Edmonton is top notch. They do great things and the people who work and volunteer there should be commended. I have an utmost respect for them all and cannot express with words my true feelings regarding them. Prior to starting treatment you have to take an introduction to the Cross session. You will get a booklet which you must read and then see a video reiterating the information in hand. It is mandatory and very useful as it opens your eyes to the various experiences you may encounter during your treatments.

It had been a few months since surgery, and as I sat there I recognized a man in the first row. It was Russell, I was sure of it. Here was the man who I had shared a hospital room with just prior to surgery. Last we met I said goodnight, the next morning I was awoken and taken to surgery never to return to that room again. In the chaos and turmoil of my situation it was a nice turn of events to see someone I sort of knew that understood a bit about what I was going through.

After the information session I worked my way through the crowd, yes that is crowd of patients, and re-introduced myself saying hello. We did some catching up and I found out he had some heart surgery after I left for my surgery, the result being he felt fantastic and much the new man. However, he elected not to have the surgery on his tumor at this time as it was located on his voice box and this meant the loss of his voice if he had done so. Our treatments were otherwise the same consisting of 30 Radiation treatments and three doses of Cysplatin Chemotherapy. We found out our start dates were the same and times of therapy were about an hour and a half part so there was a good chance of running into each other throughout our sessions. We said our goodbyes and looked forward somewhat to hooking up again during our treatments.

I met Russell in my first hospital room as I awaited surgery. He was a very social individual and we seemed to hit it off with light conversation. He had a loving beautiful new bride and what I thought of as everything to live for. He was a waiter at one of Edmonton's finest establishments and was getting set to retire in a small quiet town in Saskatchewan where he could while away the hours in peace. I think about Russell off and on as we seemed to have struck up a solid friendship that would take us through our treatments and onward via Facebook after we parted ways.

Chapter 15

Radiation

Thirty treatments of radiation were scheduled. Prior to the beginning of this you get more reading and a one on one meeting with an individual that will go through the ins and outs of what you are about to undergo. You will discuss how the treatment will be completed, how it may affect you, how it is designed for you, immediate side effects, lasting side effects and so on. It is a very comprehensive one on one and very informative to you the patient.

For my treatment I would have a plaster mold made of my face so that I could be bolted to a table, keeping my head in the same position and motionless for each treatment. The treatment would occur every day of the week around the same time except on weekends and last for about twenty minutes.

The plaster mold as I mentioned, was of my face. How they make this mold, is with two individuals working as a team, and in a little over five minutes you are done. What happens is, one talks to you and times the setting of the plaster, while the other molds the mask to your face. As I said, it only takes about five minutes to set, but it is a very long five minutes. It is a strange smothering experience and those that build it are very good at what they do.

Think of a sheet of plaster, approximately a centimeter in thickness and the size of a towel big enough to drape over your entire face, neck and shoulders allowing enough area to drape flat on the table as you lie there. This provides enough room for anchors to be put in place which will attach you to the radiation table. Now saturate the plaster sheet with water, and then drape this heavy sheet over your face with nothing but a small breathing hole for your nostrils, mouth and a couple of small holes for your eyes. To get a feel for it, I could suggest having a friend or loved one hold a pillow over your face and press down for five minutes. If you are claustrophobic this entire exercise will be one of torture which won't improve as you have the actual treatments done. I am pretty good under these conditions it turns out. I went through it uncomfortably, but none the worse for it, once it was all said and done.

The timer's job sounds simple. Watch the clock and talk you through this event while at the same time keeping you calm and motionless. The molder's job is to complete the smothering form of your face in an efficient manner so that it will be useable on the radiation table and formed perfectly to your face so it is impossible for you to move during radiation. I can't remember completely, but a laser cross hair is used to center your head and face so it is always in the exact same position every time you get bolted to the table for your treatment. Every 30 seconds the talker calls out the time, saying how fine you are doing, just a little longer, only a little while to go. In the meantime you are starting to freak out wondering if you will make it through this smothering event alive. Once it is firmly molded and set in place it is then removed and sent to the drying room. This entire exercise is done very precisely as it is not one you want to have need of repeating.

The radiation treatment itself is designed and programed by a nuclear physicist type of individual. It must be very precise as you cannot receive radiation on the same place twice I think was how the spiel went. Not sure exactly how it's administered except to say you are physically bolted to a table that slides into a round cylinder and there are lots of flashing lights and whirring and snapping sounds and even the faint smell of burning hair now and again.

Your treatment goes like this. First you check in with the radiology team and go sit in the waiting room while they load your program for you. Each day the radiation is directed with pinpoint accuracy to the adjacent spot as the previous day's appointment. This is all controlled by the computer program set up for you by the nuclear physicist type guy. How this works is beyond my capabilities of imagination, but suffice to say, it does work.

Second you get escorted into the room where you are asked your name again and birthdate then assisted to lie down on the table as they place the mold over your face and bolt your head and shoulders to the table. Once bolted in place, the table is slid into the cylinder machine whereas a laser cross hair is lined up with the cross hair markings on your mask perfectly and the table is locked into place. The radiation technologist then turns on the machine and leaves the room to the safety of another room. Here they can watch you on a TV screen, and talk to you if need be, through a speaker radio system.

Thirdly the machine starts doing its thing, you lie there on the table in your gown for fifteen or twenty minutes alone, peaking out of the holes in your mask. Again I reiterate, not a happy place for claustrophobic peoples. My treatment was complicated with the nausea created by chemotherapy. Imagine being put into the position of being bolted down on your back to a table in a mask and needing to vomit with your nearest help in the next room and you helplessly bolted down. The mask doesn't just pop off in a second. You have to make a muffled cry for help to show that you are in distress and wait for the radiation machine to shut down so it is safe for them to enter and unbolt you. Hopefully, you aren't choking to death but the breathing holes were quite small so I am thinking it is a real possibility. These thoughts have a way of making a person feel anxious.

On bad nausea days treatment was cancelled because I couldn't hold anything down and was too scared to lie on my back let alone allow someone to bolt me down to a table. On my better days I would lie back and try to calm my mind. One thing that worked out for me was my love for music and the soothing sounds of Pink Floyd, Dark Side of the Moon to be specific. No, you can't bring your IPod into the machine with you. Although it would be nice if they had a system in future that would allow you more comfort. You could maybe choose some relaxing music for whenever your treatment is running and they could pipe it through the sound system as background music to listen to if you so desired. Seems like an easy thing to accomplish. That said, I have listened to that album hundreds of times over the years to relax me and float away. So as I searched my mind for calming influences as I was bolted to the table, I came across the album and begun to play it in my mind from start to finish. I could play just about a complete side and actually would drift off to sleep some days as I lay there. It is important to find something solid and calming to grab hold of while you are in there. It may take some time, but once you find it, you will find you tolerate the entire experience better.

During your various treatments and therapies, learn to tolerate, and I would suggest allowing students to learn from your case. In radiation one day, they were training a new technologist to run the machine. You have to learn by doing eventually so have patience. This particular day was her first time at running it, and I was one of her first patients, if not her very first patient and you could sense she was nervous. She was aware that these masks and such are not the most comfortable setups, so she was trying to be as caring and efficient as possible. She bolted me down and struggled to get the machine lined up, but with the help of her trainer she got me ready to go and we were on are way or so I thought. She then accidentally hit the wrong button which halted the entire process making it so that the machine would require a warm up and realignment again prior to my treatment being started. This entire time I spent bolted quietly in my mask to the table. By the time we were finished, 45 minutes had passed by and she was mortified. Once I left the radiation room I found my Mother freaking out in a panic in the waiting room, mad as hell, wondering about what had occurred. I was ok having slept through half of it so be patient and accepting that mistakes happen, this is a stressful time for not only you but your care provider to.

Chapter 16

Hair Loss

What does a cancer patient look like? I suppose if you try and picture it in your mind a stereotypical view would be that of an individual with most if not all of their hair fallen out, looking deathly ill, as if they had just been saved from the death grips of a concentration camp in World War II. This however is not always the case. I for example, much to the disappointment of the many balding friends I have, did not lose my hair. Only some chemotherapies cause baldness. This was a dream come true in a bad situation as far as my vanity and self-consciousness were concerned, but it also allowed for some levity in the situation. This allowed the jokes to fly with regards to hair loss giving me something to laugh about and then it helped my own view of self in the mirror. Some days were hard enough to look in the mirror with the scars both visible and hidden as it is. I didn't need the added burden of losing all my hair.

Chapter 17

Chemo – First Dose

Chemotherapy can be defined as bringing you to the edge of death by poison and then pulling you back, just before you cross the point of no return and venture into the great unknown. Sometimes you might just wish that you fell over the precipice. Just remember that once you return from the voyage and see all that you love before you, it will be worth it. There is nothing that is as precious as life itself and all the glories that come with it.

Prior to my first dose I had an appointment with the Doctor who would be overseeing my chemotherapy. He explained to me some of the side effects of the drug and described the cycle of ups and downs my immune system would encounter throughout the treatment. He gave me a symptom tracking card that I was to fill out every day of my therapy to identify and track physical and mental issues that I was experiencing. Such things as nausea, how many times had you vomited today, could you eat solids, or just clear liquids and so on. I was to receive three doses in total, one every two weeks. He gave me a letter to hand to a hospital emergency, if I had certain extreme reactions that may be fatal or very serious at any rate they could refer to the letter and call him if need be. I took this time to ask the question I had on my mind. I had thought about it on many occasions but had been avoiding and never broached with any other Doctor. It was, "What is my chance of survival?" I asked it. His reply was, "43%". I stated, "So I am batting five hundred" and he stated, "No, not quite." Now I understand that his world revolves around pure data of research and statistical analysis. Also, I can appreciate being brutally honest and straight up to your patients, but instead of not quite, maybe the words, yes almost, may have been more uplifting to me as a patient trying to make it through this.

What a day and what a night. My first dose of chemotherapy was a day I will never forget. It started with a little bit of anxiety, wondering how my body would react. Would I survive? Was I going to have a bad reaction? Or, would it be ok? I arrived to my appointment early, in order to get it over with as soon as possible. The wait was driving me crazy. My treatment consisted of being hooked up to an IV bag for about an hour or so. This time went by uneventful. I was made very comfortable receiving a blanket freshly out of the warmer to snuggle under and drift off if I so desired. I would suggest always bringing a good book when you go for your treatments as one hour can sometimes become one or two hours wait time plus another hour hooked up to your IV. Sometimes delays occur so just be patient and tolerant, you will get your poison eventually.

So my first treatment was working its way through my system, ready to do battle with the Cancer. I left the Cross Cancer Clinic feeling happy and confident that this wasn't so bad. I could handle this no problem. I went home to my parents and joined them in a nice meal. Still feeling great after dinner I thought this would be a good time to hook up for an evening of some good conversation with an old friend. I told my parents my intention and called my buddy to see if he was available. He was, so I hopped in my car and headed over. Over the years we have had many an enjoyable evening sitting downstairs having a couple beers and shooting the breeze as we watch a hockey game or play a little online poker. This evening was no exception and went off without a hitch. I had been through one hell of a battle over the past months and stated matter of fact like. Let's have a beer. I figured this was a treat for all the suffering I had experienced, and I was feeling pretty good about myself so why not. It took me about two hours to sip and swallow my way through that beer but it was enjoyable and that's what counted.

About eleven o'clock that night I started to feel a wave of fatigue come over me and I asked if I could go lie down. He said no problem, so off I went to the spare room to sleep for the night. Exhausted and feeling satisfied with my day I started to doze off. Next thing I know, I was not feeling very good anymore and felt that any moment I was going to vomit. I hurried down the hall and made it, just on time. Anything that was in my stomach revolted and was now gone. This continued about every half hour to 45 minutes throughout the night. After the second time my stomach was pretty much voided of all that was in it and the dry heaves commenced. My stomach convulsed and wretched, it was pure agony. Strange that in this position I felt bad for keeping my friend and his family awake all night. I must have vomited a dozen times by morning. My radiation appointment was around 10 AM that day I think, and I was in no shape to drive so my buddy took me to the Cross for my appointment. What normally would have been a twenty minute drive ended up stretched out as we were forced to pull over three times so I could hang my head into the gutter expelling what I could.

My perspective is that chemotherapy is like picking your own special poison. The objective of chemotherapy is to kill the Cancer. The easiest way to do this as I stated earlier is by bringing you to the brink of death and then pulling you back just before you fall off the edge. You see the worse it makes you feel is a measure in its success fighting the Cancer, because it is having the same effect on the Cancer in your body.

I think this is where the saying came from, what doesn't kill you, will make you stronger. Ask a chemotherapist and they will say yes I am trying to kill you, almost, and twenty years ago it was more like you would end up dead from the cure most of the time. Maybe, I exaggerate here but not by very much, this is the real deal. My dosage had to be reduced as I was encountering an extreme reaction. Good thing they sent me home with all those in case of a medical emergency letters and numbers, and a very good thing they had a nurse on call waiting for a person like me to phone and say things are not going very well and I feel like I am going to die. So much for the couple hundred dollars spent on miracle anti-nausea medications.

So what happens to all these destroyed cancer cells. Well the movie Alien comes to mind but the little star of the show doesn't make an appearance by ripping a hole in your stomach, but where he does come out isn't very nice and should be listed as toxic waste. If you weren't religious before this event you may be after it.

Chapter 18

Can't Drive Anymore

The same stubbornness that kept me alive to this point was almost my undoing. They do not do radiation on the weekends so I tried to go home to my kids in Drayton Valley after my first Chemo experience. My ex, my parents, and my friends all offered to drive me the hour and a half back into the city for my treatments but I said "No, I can make it, I will be fine" I had been puking for days now, unable to hold down anything for very long that I did manage to eat. I couldn't even hold water. Dehydrated and weakened by it all I headed out. Clothes bag in the back seat, big paper grocery bag filled with used Kleenex on the passenger seat beside me. I was still going through massive amounts of Kleenex, continually trying to clear my throat of the rope like saliva in my throat and wiping my constantly runny nose.

About 30 kilometers down the highway I felt the rush of nausea. It was all I could do to stop myself hurling all over the dash of the car. I immediately pulled to the shoulder simultaneously grabbing for the big paper grocery bag and spewed all what was bad inside me. This act was repeated another half dozen times before reaching my destination and the safety of my parent's home. After the third or fourth time I was starting to rethink my decision about the drive and berate myself for being so pig headed and stupid. This however did not change the simple fact that I still had to complete the drive. I was committed now, to what I had started, and couldn't just give in. It was one thing to know myself that I had screwed up and bitten off more than I could chew but this was not something I could mention to any of those that had offered to help me. The words, I told you so, were already ringing in my ears. This was a very hard trip indeed and it would be the last one which I would be driving for a long time.

It is hard to lose your independence, but when you are putting yourself as well as others on the road at risk it is just not worth it. People care for you and do not consider it as an imposition on them to help you in any way possible. It is not a sign of weakness to ask for a helping hand, it is a sign of strength. I cannot say this enough. They truly want to help, and I think in some regards it helps them deal with your situation better because it gives them an opportunity to do something towards your recovery rather than sit helpless on the sidelines watching you fight it alone. I think it is a very helpless feeling when you watch someone you care about struggle and there is nothing you can do to ease their pain.

Chapter 19

Parents Moving

Life must go on around you whether you are sick or not. What should have been a positive welcome time in my parent's life became one filled with stress and worry. In the middle of my chemo and radiation treatments my parents were successful in the selling of their old house and the purchase of their dream retirement condo.

It was a time they should have welcomed. A time of no more lawn mowing, snow shoveling, or major exterior home maintenance to look forward to. It was a time to enjoy the sweeter things in life. Having worked so hard so long and reap the benefits of a long career to focus on themselves for a change. This was not to be. They had a son to work around in the move. I was too weak to do much else other then get in the way. Moving unto itself is stressful enough. Imagine doing this at the same time your housing your adult child, who many think, including maybe you, won't see his next birthday. It must be almost unbearable.

I would ask them myself to see how this felt to them at the time, but it is much too raw and real still at this time to discuss. I don't think I could handle it. All those emotions brought back to the surface. One day maybe, perhaps after they get to read this book, but not now.

My sister was a life saver. The tension at my parent's house was extreme. Something had to give as the boiling point was close to being reached between them. The possession date was approaching and it was time to move me out. Weighing in at 152 pounds and having experienced a loss of over 70 pounds so far, there wasn't much of me to move. They packed up my medications and bag of clothes and off I went to my sisters.

Chapter 20

PEG Tube 1 – The Death Camp Look

As I said, my fighting weight was down to 152 lbs. I had lost the battle and was losing the war fast. At the next appointment I had with my Radiation Doctor, I discussed the dreaded feeding tube. To me this was like giving up. It was a very depressing thought imagining going through life with a feeding tube implanted into your stomach. I didn't like this idea at all, but knew if I was to have any chance of survival this was it. I think I am very strong willed and stubborn you might say. I had not learned a thing from my driving incident as I vomited my way into the city. There is a time to ask for help. I just about missed mine. Just make sure you don't ask when it is too late as I almost did.

My body had taken a beating. The chemotherapy was in full swing and I was well into the radiation treatments. Although I felt in pretty good shape after the surgery, the reality was my body was still directing energy to heal itself and in repair mode. I was basically consuming myself, but had reached a state where I had no reserves left to consume. I think it is safe to say that it wasn't looking like I would be in the 43% survival group of the statistics. More now than ever, it was very likely I now fell into the "fatal majority" category of the numbers game before me.

Prior to an evaluation with the Doctor who would install the PEG Tube, he stated, that he would only perform the procedure if there was a bed for me at the Cross Cancer Institute to which my Radiation Specialist said there would be. I was weak, beaten down and ready to give up. I thought it was the only way I stood a chance of surviving, a magic bullet so to speak, and a reprieve.

I was put under and the procedure went on without a hitch. I even got pictures to take home afterwards showing the view as the camera and light went down into my throat. First you could see the graft from my arm. It was very strange indeed. A pale white looking bit of flesh in the back of my throat with a couple of hairs growing out of it. I guess now if I get a tickle in my throat I have some explanations. Then down towards my stomach it went, shining the light ahead of it. I guess what happens is the light can be seen on the outside of your stomach through your skin, just like when you put a flashlight under your hand camping. They line it up on the inside and this reddish glow marks where to cut on the outside of your stomach. I am guessing here, but then they cut the hole and the tube becomes held in place by an open umbrella end of plastic material on the inside so that it doesn't fall out of the hole in your stomach. Then a bit is slid down the tube on the outside to hold it firmly in place to both sides of your skin. You spin the tube daily to ensure that it doesn't heal completely and weld to your flesh. In this way it is possible to remove without cutting again, if you reach a stage where you are not dependent on it for nutrition anymore.

I think this was a Thursday or Friday and after the surgery I went home to my sister's house and awaited the call for my room at the Cross. The hospital had sent us away with some rations and instructions on how to maintain and do the tube feeds so I would be alright for a few days. My sister hung the bag, much like an IV, off her curtain rod and there we were set up with a gravity feed system. My new rubber umbilical cord or life line was in place.

One day's wait became two, then the weekend passed us by and Monday my sister took me to my radiation treatment at the Cross hoping they would have some answers and some new accommodations for me. She dropped me off at the front door to the building and I gathered up all my strength and walked the little way to the registration desk just inside the main doors. There was a small line ahead of me. As I stood waiting, I started to waiver on my feet. I thought to myself, there is no way I am falling. I am not going to be pushed around in a wheel chair like some helpless invalid. What a complete idiot I was. There I stood, life hanging by a thread and I was still too stubborn to enjoy a free ride on a wheel chair like it was beneath me and wimpy. How irrational is that? Some tough guy I was, fool more like. It didn't have to be this way. I didn't have to do everything the hard way, but I guess that's just how I am wired. Who knows, maybe this idiocy is what saved me in the long run. I was just too dumb to die, and not smart enough to give up.

The line was going deathly slow. Standing was so hard. My body was going to let me down, but my mind pulled it onward. Just when I thought I was going to have to cry out for help and collapse, the line ended and it was my turn. I moved forward, crossing the red tape line on the floor and gave the receptionist my little red card. Name and birthdate she asked. I told her, in my hoarse whisper of a voice and waited for my orders. She printed them off and sent me on my way to radiation. Jen had returned, car parked, and ready to get some answers. I gathered myself again and off we went down the escalator to radiation and my next treatment.

Turns out the Doctor who had installed my PEG Tube was in my corner that day and had checked into my room situation. Upset to hear that I wasn't in a room yet, he pursued it further and resolved this issue. I would not be seeing the outside of the building for the foreseeable future. It was convenient in many ways. Lifting the burden of my care from my family and putting it in the hands of professionals. It was also an eye opener to just what kind of situation I was in. It was a sobering reality check.

Now since I had not known I was going to be having a sleep over for some time I did not bring anything but me. They booked me into my room and my sister headed home to get what belongings I had that would make my stay a little more comfortable. Toothpaste, my favorite comforter blanket, books to keep me human and occupy my mind. Then, she set me up with a television rental to help while away the hours. While she was gone a nurse came in and hooked me up for my tube feed of the day. I was informed that the volume of intake would be set at a minimum level for fear of shocking my system. One tablespoon every fifteen minutes or something as outrageous sounding as that it was. I wasn't aware at the time, but you can shock a body to death with food within the first few days of resuming intake after starving it for so long. I guess it makes sense once explained. As close as I can find for an explanation of this, is a description of Refeeding Syndrome. This is to say, any individual who has had negligible nutrient intake for five consecutive days is at risk of this syndrome.

Once feeding resumes, the worst case scenario is that the potential exists for fatal cardiac arrhythmias. I hadn't eaten in eleven days with the exception of some liquids in an IV bag until the PEG Tube was installed.

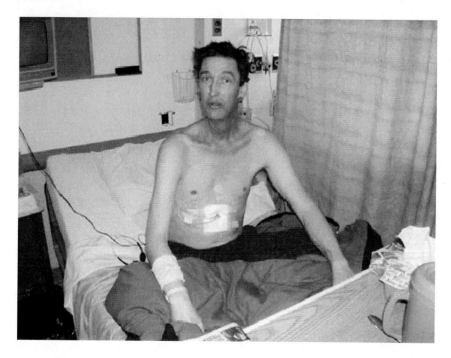

So I am very thankful that I did not go into convulsions, coma or cardiac arrest while in the care of my sister. I just couldn't imagine what that would be like for a sibling to encounter. Looking back now, the common theme seems to be; how did I survive that one? Over, and over again it amazes me how resilient the body is, and how powerful the mind can be. I can only hope people can learn from my errors in judgment and that they do not need to make it this hard for themselves.

Chapter 21

Stay at the Cross

This time is very fragmented. I have little bits and pieces of various memories here and there. Some memories I try to block out, and others are in a fog that I cannot quite grasp. There I sat. Seventy to eighty pounds lighter (30 to 35 kilos lighter) looking scared and frail, the strength in me gone.

Although nourishment and survival were my main concerns here, I still continued daily radiation and now weekly chemo treatments of a lesser strength dose. You do not get a room in this facility unless you are at risk. This was a harsh reality which was becoming clear to me. As soon as you are off the danger list you are out the door and your bed is freed up to put some other poor soul in it. I think I spent a couple of weeks in their special care and I hold a deep respect and admiration for those who work and volunteer for the patients and their families day in, day out. I could not do it. My heart couldn't take it. Many of the patients they deal with will never see outside those walls again, I am one of the lucky ones. My treatment was first class in every manner possible and it is not one I will ever forget.

So there I was, literally starving to death and given a new chance to survive by this second belly button so to speak. A rubber umbilical cord, hooked up to a bag of liquid life. It had all the nutrients I required for a proper diet. Mm mm, vanilla flavored burps brought back the not so sweet memories, of a nasal feeding tube from a time not too distant gone.

Starvation brings with it many complications. I hadn't eaten for over a week other then maybe a little bit of tomato soup, nothing with any solid food sustenance in it anyway. What happened to me is my digestive system for lack of use started to shut down and things were not working very well so to speak. With my new food intake directly to the stomach via my PEG Tube the entry was taken care of, but since there had been no exit in many days, things were not flowing at all well. Morphine has a way of compounding this issue with one of its side effects, as it creates blockage issues.

All my life, gas, number two events, and issues related to them, had been the brunt or source of many endless jokes but this was no laughing matter now. Every day the nurse came into the room and asked matter of fact like; how many days since your last bowel movement? Once we hit three, it was out of my hands so to speak and time to jump into action. Now throughout my ordeal my pride and dignity took small beatings here and there. Being too weak to bath myself, I couldn't wash my hair, having my mom feed me were all examples of this. This time it was just too much. It has pained me for hours just to figure out a way to write this. I really struggled with even including it, but finally came to the conclusion with the help of my girlfriend that I have to tell the whole story if it is to take on full value to anyone that follows in preparation for what may be to come.

I was not left with a shred of dignity to hang on to by the end of this affair. Day three came and went uneventful, no movements to speak of. It was time to act and in came the nurse that evening with a big syringe full of laxative to fire into the feeding tube. Hopeful that it would soon be over and normalcy would once more be in my grasp, I went to sleep. Next morning nothing became of it. The nurse came in and asked those now dreaded words, how many days since your last bowel movement. Four days I answered. More laxative was the solution and more was given. Continued feeding, still no relief. Pressure continued to build. Stress, discomfort and pain combined to produce misery now. This problem was not going away and the nursing staff was going to deal with it until it was resolved. Utter and complete humiliation would hardly express how I was feeling at the time.

I had to go, my guts roiled in pain, off to the bathroom I went time and time again with the same lack of result. It was late afternoon now of day four and my mother came to visit while I was on a trip to the bathroom. I tried and tried to no avail. It was like trying to shift a cement plug, no chance. One hour went by, closing in on two hours I still sat in that little room my mother outside the door waiting by my bedside. I couldn't go and it was hurting now.

I hit the nurse alert from in the bathroom and explained my predicament. To her this was just part of a normal day. To me this was the end of my world, the last bit, or so I thought, of dignity stripped from me. Back she came a few minutes later knocking at the door. Time for the next step she said, and showed me a suppository. Wishing this would be my salvation I obliged her and hoped. Time ticked by and there I sat and stood and sat on and on. Finally humiliated, exhausted and frustrated I exited the bathroom and lay down. I just wanted sleep to take me. I didn't want to be part of this world no more. My mom said her goodbyes and left me to rest.

A short while later another nurse arrived. She was a little more senior then the others and had dealt with troubled cases similar to this in the past I am sure. She quietly explained to me the final solution and how she was confident my problems would soon be over. I would be flushed out so to speak and off she went to gather what she needed. Professionally she was fantastic. I could sense her empathy and if it were not for the circumstances that we were in would have considered her quite motherly and gentle. She administered the treatment and quietly left explaining how once I felt it working I was to go to the bathroom and ring the nurse's call button.

The moment I felt anything, my abdominal cavity clenched and went into extreme convulsions and I was racked with pain. I couldn't sit up let alone walk, there was no way out. I cried out in agony for help, but none was to be had, and evacuated my insides. The pain was excruciating but once complete relieving. I couldn't do anything but look away from my doorway at the divider wall in my room and hit the nurse's button for assistance as instructed. There I lay in my own filth, degraded, humiliated and crying in a whimper. I truly wanted to die. The embarrassment was too great to take. She came in quietly and saw me laying there motionless, dignity completely destroyed and went to work. Within minutes all traces of those events were gone and replaced with fresh linens and bed clothes. She understood the trauma I had just experienced and I felt her compassion. She allowed me to be quiet, alone in my hell, not having to acknowledge the reality through conversation. I thank her very much for allowing me this as without it I couldn't have faced another day.

Now I sit broken, in my chair typing, still wondering if I can handle the embarrassment of it all. Friends, family and strangers alike knowing my most private memories, bared to the world for all to see and judge.

Sometimes I wonder what I did in my life that was so bad I deserved this outcome, and curse my existence for it. Other times I am proud that I am so strong to take this burden and live through it, so that I may share it and make the life of hopefully one person more bearable because of it.

Chapter 22

Lemon Meringue Pie

Radiation and chemo treatment finished, my reward for surviving hell on earth for the six months previous was a lemon meringue pie. It is one of my favorite things. A delicious desert that I thought, all things considered would go down easy. Even if I couldn't eat the crust, the filling and topping should have gone down nice and easy, sliding down my throat was my thinking. There was just one little thing I forgot about, and that was the after effects of the radiation treatments on my mouth and throat.

Once my thirty treatments were completed, the radiation continued to do its work, burning its way through me for a couple more weeks. What happened in my case was that my throat and mouth started blistering from the treatments and open sores could be found throughout.

The pie looked so good, but I had forgotten that lemons have a special way about them. The affect being a burning stinging sensation which was felt on every open wound within my mouth and throat as that great delight made its way to my stomach. It was agony, I almost cried, pure delicious agony. I continued as long as I could but soon it became unbearable and I had to give up on the dream. Eventually I would be able to eat that pie, but that day was still a ways off. Looking back now, all I can say is what an idiot I was and laugh.

Chapter 23

Starting to Rehabilitate and Recover

I didn't really have a voice to speak of. I had my little white board to write on and if someone was close enough I could whisper to them quietly in a hoarse raspy way. To some, such as my son on the soccer field, this was heaven on earth, finally a little peace and quiet where I was concerned. There I sat day in day out, too weak and frail to move much. Laptop by my side, the TV remote within reach, and the IV stand for my PEG Tube feedbag close by. Skin and bone and sitting on a big soft leather couch for hours on end.

It was strange not having a voice as the world ran around me. An ordinary day went something like this. Between 0230 and 0300 AM I would wake up and wonder why I was wide awake. I would lay there staring at the ceiling for a good hour usually just waiting for a sleep that never came. Once my hope ran out, I would reach over and grab my laptop. Then proceed to play some free poker tournaments online that would hopefully burn a couple of hours for me. If I was really good and lucky that night, I would play for about three hours and sometimes win a prize of a couple dollars or an entry to another tournament. I enjoyed this cheap entertainment because it whiled away the hours, and didn't take much effort other than a mouse click, but yet it kept my mind engaged.

Usually a wave of exhaustion would start to hit about 0500AM or so and it would be time to sleep. Sometimes I would pass out while playing and wake with my laptop next to me and the game although long over, still on. In my condition, my neck and arms were not very conducive to holding a book in my hands for reading long stretches of time without discomfort. Having this outlet as an alternative was very welcome indeed, because in order to pull your body along your mind must be energized and sharp.

About 1000AM my body would stir and with great effort I would pull it off the bed. This was itself a great accomplishment because it felt so heavy and weighted down. Each day I would have to tell my body to lift itself. Some days I just couldn't do it, so I would sort of roll off the side of the bed as controlled as possible and once semi kneeling on the floor I would pull myself to standing using the bed as support.

Then up the basement stairs I would go, using my hands on the steps above to help me, in search of my first medications of the day. For the first while I had quite the selection of meds. There were about ten different varieties to navigate through. This is where some of the benefits of research come to pass. One such researcher was doing a thesis regarding setting up excel spreadsheet medicine schedules for patients and the value of doing so. I signed up and he organized my meds on a simple spreadsheet. It was very convenient because there were so many. Some had to be taken at different times than others. Some needed to be taken at meal time and some on an empty stomach. This gets to be a little unsettling when you have so many to keep track of and are in the midst of self-administering morphine every four to six hours. Having a schedule insured all medication was taken at the appropriate time and not missed.

Since my swallow was compromised, pills were very hard to get down. They constantly would get stuck in my throat and on more than one occasion the only way I managed to free them was to vomit them out. Part of the reason for this was that the anatomy in my throat and mouth had been altered forever and part of it was that most of my saliva glands were destroyed by the radiation treatments. Any saliva I did have was thick and ropey and hard to shift. Sticky and much like glue. The way I describe my swallow if you want to experience a similar condition to it, is this. Think of a day when you were parched and your mouth was dry as a bone. You got that thought in your head now. Ok, even without that reality, walk over to the cupboard in your kitchen or even run out to the store and get a half dozen premium plus crackers. Now without anything to wash them down, put those six crackers in your mouth and try to swallow them down. Is there a problem? Come on swallow them for me. There you go, fun isn't it. You just walked a mile in my shoes.

Most of the pills I would crush and syringe them down with water into my PEG Tube. That said, I should mention that my ex and my kids did this most days for me initially as I didn't have the strength to crush them myself. Once the pills were in me it was time to head off to the bathroom to gargle or at the very least swish warm water clumsily in my mouth. This moisture in my dry mouth, with a tongue I did not know how to work and the thick ropey saliva pasted against the walls of my mouth and throat was a necessary evil. It would just plain and simple, aggravate the situation, and make me cough and wheeze. The moisture would bind to some of the saliva making it glue like, so that it threatened to choke me as I attempted to swallow or clear it from my airways. Having the constant feeling of being choked is not a pleasant thing. It was very uncomfortable and I would cough, and cough and cough harder to try to shift it and rid my throat of its misery. It was next to impossible some days to expel. I would get it half way out where I almost had it gone and lose it. Then I would have to manually pull out those slimy ropes by hand, one at a time, reaching in and gagging all the way. A gross and unpleasant misery, it was. Usually I would cough and cough until I vomited; finally clearing my throat of any remnants and this morning ritual would allow me comfort at last. The ability to breathe normally once again without fear or the constant feeling I was going to choke to death. Then off to the couch I went to hook up to my lifeline of liquid food to my stomach tube.

This would take about an hour to run through at which time the children would soon be home for lunch from school sometimes with friends. My youngest boy David seemed impressed by it all, so he would bring home a friend to show my scars off to and such so the day sometimes had a few funny moments in it all. After lunch time the house would fall quiet again and there I would be sitting watching the TV. Luckily for me there was world class soccer to watch in the afternoon, until the bell rang in the distance signaling the days end at school.

Often the phone would ring, and at first my initial reaction was to hurry to it as fast as I could and say hello. The thing was, I didn't move very fast and when I said hello, I wasn't loud enough for anyone on the other end to hear me. So after a couple of times answering out of habit I would just sit and listen to it ring.

Pain for me came from many areas, just sitting hurt. I didn't have full blown bed sores but was pretty raw in some areas. My muscle tissue had wasted away to almost nothing more than thin ropes like a puppets strings maneuvering my body here and there. The muscle deterioration was so great you could see muscles on my back that under normal circumstances would have never been seen and would have been buried from view by layers of outer muscles. I controlled the pain with my mickey of morphine, administering a good dose into my stomach tube as the pain started to become unbearable.

The kids would arrive at the end of the day and I would just feel happy to watch them go about their daily routines. With them came an energy that I could feed off of. A joyous moment in an otherwise lonely painful existence filled with staring at the walls.

After a few days homecare started to make an appearance and then came physiotherapy at the hospital which got me motivated to start walking and building my strength slowly. It took me quite a while to build up to it but soon I was walking for a good hour each day. I started slow. First I went a couple houses down the street then turned around. Once I got to half a block I kept pushing and tried to go all the way around the block. There was a bench about ¾ of the way around and I sat down to rest and ready myself to push on. Soon I was walking to the hospital and back then venturing out around town planning my route so that I made sure I had available rest stops along the way. I made sure I had Kleenex with me everywhere to clear my throat and wipe my nose. My nose ran continuously it seemed. This always struck me as strange because I had no saliva but I seemed to have an endless nasal drip. No cold to speak of, just a runny nose. By the end of the summer I could walk five kilometers, pretty good by anyone's standards I would say.

Once the blisters started to disappear, my voice slowly started to come back. The trache was long gone, and the swelling and blisters associated with my radiation treatments had dissipated. There I sat talking in a whisper at most and now it was time to eat.

Sitting on the steps watching the world go by at this time, was my idea of heaven. No need to use my challenged voice or work at chewing, just sit and watch time pass by. The thing was, it was something I just couldn't do. I had lost so much weight so fast that my muscle mass had wasted away to nothing. It was like sitting on bone and painful to the point where I could not even sit down on the concrete stairs to tie my shoes. All semblance of padding on my butt had disappeared, I was a walking skeleton.

Physiotherapy is a long winded necessary evil. You get out of it what you put into it. Don't expect miracles in the first week because you will just disappoint yourself. When I started out I was doing curls with a one pound can of soup and I could feel the burn after a few reps of ten I tell you.

Back to walking I went, one foot in front of the other. I used to go to my son's soccer practice and walk laps as they practiced. I started slowly and worked myself up as I went. If I got tired, I just sat down and rested watching them play or run a drill. Slowly I got better and would sit behind the net to catch balls and kick them back if they flew over the net. Again baby steps, I would walk to the ball and slowly dribble it back then kick it to the goalie. After a few weeks I built up some leg strength and managed to boot the ball pretty good. I couldn't run but I was on the mend.

Chapter 24

Warfarin and Cardio-Version

Warfarin, otherwise known as rat poison, is a heavy duty blood thinner and was a real treat to be on. Earlier I mentioned the small complication that was found regarding arrhythmias or an irregular heartbeat and it was now time to deal with it. I was now up to about 168 lbs. and recovered to some extent.

I could walk about five kilometers in a 45 minute period and was starting to feel strong again. The purpose of the warfarin was to regulate the blood consistency to reduce the potential for clots.

When they give you a cardio version, what they do is knock you out and then hit you with the paddles, to shock your heart into a regular beat. That said, the shock interrupts the hearts natural beat and stops it to some degree then lets the blood flow again with a contraction. My understanding is that when this contraction occurs, it pushes the blood through your system releasing clots that may exist if you have not been pre- treated with blood thinners. This treatment with Warfarin, can last for weeks and sometimes months, prior to the procedure being done.

When they say blood thinner, they mean it. Keep all sharp objects away and don't shave with a manual razor for fear of nicking yourself. Any cuts including the pin-hole left by giving blood samples or IVs and are very tough to clot. When you get your Warfarin, you get a nice kit and card that you keep with you in case of an accident where you are bleeding. This way the paramedics or emerge staff know they have to work fast to control the bleeding. Comforting isn't it? A bit dramatic, but real nevertheless. This wasn't my problem with the whole warfarin thing though, my problem was the twice a week lab test.

Twice a week I wandered over to the lab and got blood work done to measure if I was in the proper range and stable enough I my numbers to get my cardio version completed with the least amount of risk to me. In the past I had never had a problem with needles. I even used to watch them put the needle in and draw out whatever amounts they needed. I am forever changed now and feel so wimpy for it but I understand where it comes from.

There was a time through my treatments when I was receiving at least 10 needles a day for pain, taking blood samples, and administering various meds. I was fine through all this. Then veins started collapsing and running to hide from the needles. It took one nurse seven times to get an IV in me one day. She started with the usual inner arm areas and quickly went to the veins on my hand. I looked like a pin cushion and felt bad for her. After the first couple she was feeling bad about hurting me, but I was numb to it by that time so I felt bad for her. After recovering from this stay in the hospital and being home for a while without any needles required, I had become a little shell shocked of it all. Now I had to look forward to this twice a week. I cringed at every needle, whether they hurt or not, and still shy away to this day. I look away every time and cringe at the thought of it piercing my skin.

One thing I did learn that may provide some comfort for you is that there are different sizes of needles and if they use a finer one it hurts less. I appreciate the lab tech telling me this as it has alleviated some of the grief I feel when I go for any blood work now. I mention it when I go to the lab sometimes and request that they use a finer needle if possible and sometimes luck out.

Finally stable in the optimum area of blood consistency I was off for my cardio version. It was a fairly uneventful procedure for me. Up early and then put to sleep for the actual event, I awoke a few hours later feeling fine and hungry. I felt well enough to take in the Edmonton Grande Prix race that afternoon. It was as if I had just taken a nice long nap. It was a success they told me. I had been shocked into normalcy. As we know however, nothing in life is for sure or forever and a few weeks later I reverted to my old irregular beat where I am today. I guess I really do beat to my own drum as many have suggested over the years. Not a problem though, I feel good unless I really push hard like running up a mountainside or hustling down the soccer pitch. Neither of which are not in my immediate future, maybe one day though never say never, so it's all good.

Chapter 25

Going Back to Work Full Time

Sometimes I think of this time as my "What was I thinking?" phase. Had I completely lost my mind? I truly wonder about this. Here I was eleven months after my seventeen hours of surgery, five months since the end of my thirty radiation treatments and chemotherapy, and a little over three months since my cardio-version to regulate my heart beat on my way to work fulltime again. It was November so there were not a lot of wildfires to worry about, and this time was for paperwork and training so I thought I could handle it. The people I worked with worried about me constantly. I felt exhausted most of the time. But they were very supportive and allowed me some flexibility to come in late on occasion when I needed the extra rest. My duties were modified and slowly I took on a full role again looking after my programs.

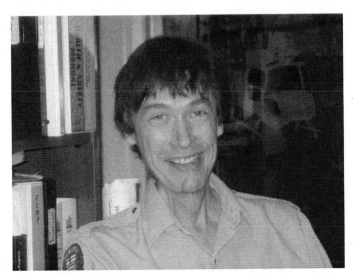

It felt good to be back at work. My weight had stabilized at 168 pounds but it was still taking me over three hours a day to chew and swallow three square meals. I still required 3000 calories a day to keep me on the mend and my lunch hour took the entire hour to swallow most days. I must have been a strange sight to see in the lunch room day in day out. The plan was, with that calorie intake, I should be able to gain a pound every one or two weeks.

Christmas Dinner 2008 was delicious, but a lot of work. Mine consisted of a small plate which was full, but not loaded down with what I would consider the monster normal portions of the past. Different foods have different textures and consistencies. This provides challenges in the different ways of grinding the food down and swallowing of each variety. In the past I would have piled as much food on my plate as it would carry and just shovel the glory of a meal down my gullet in record time running back for seconds. This day I had to keep the different textures separate and take one small bite size piece at a time chewing it until finely ground and timing a swallow with a drink to help wash it down my throat in one shot. Each small bite took a minute in duration with extra time for turkey, ham or stuffing soaked in gravy. Within half an hour the table had emptied out with the exception of me. Twenty minutes or so later the cleanup crew started to do the dishes and clean up all the potential leftovers and empty dishes from around me. I just kept grabbing drink after drink and chewing my heart out. Family members kept asking me if I would like it heated up but I just shook my head and continued on with my work. Three hours went by and there I sat finally satisfied with a clean plate before me. That was the biggest meal I had tackled in over a year and oh so good. Every minute was spent savoring the flavor and in pure bliss. It was a great accomplishment that I wanted to share with my swallow therapist and dietician. A small plate with a modest portion of dessert left me ready to join the crowd again.

I had a choice, to do the work, eat and get on with living or take the easy way out, give up the fight and get a meal out of a can one drop at a time for the rest of my life. Mm, vanilla flavored liquid or an open buffet. I chose life and the open buffet. That said, there were many foods at this time that I could not eat due to difficulty in swallowing or extreme effort in chewing. Bread and its doughy consistency once it's chewed, was impossible for me to swallow at this time. It would turn into a doughy ball and get lodged in my throat choking me. I would avoid bread at all costs. We would order pizza sometimes and I would eat the topping and leave the entire crust for fear of choking on the dough. This hurt as I loved my sandwiches, it is amazing how many meals bread or dough is a part of in everyday life.

Another favorite was beef steak. I do love beef steak, Alberta beef cannot be beat but it is something I just could not do. Ground beef was fine, and if I really really wanted I am sure I could cut the steak very small and chew it down eventually. The thing with beef steak is the texture and grain of the meat is one of the toughest around to grind down by chewing. The only way I can swallow is to grind my food into a powder almost and then wash it down with a small drink. By the time I finished a small piece of even stew meat that was crock potted all day and falling apart on the plate my teeth would hurt. The fibers in the meat were still too long and would still require mastication prior to me swallowing them down without choking.

The months to follow were spent trying different foods and seeing which would allow me the most calories with the least amount of effort in chewing while still allowing me some variety. It is amazing how dominated by diet and low calorie food the market is nowadays. I go to a smoothie counter and ask for the highest calorie one they have and they look at me like I am not all there. Go to the grocery store and you are inundated by calorie wise this, diet this, lose weight by eating this products. Eating was a very involved process you might say.

For this first while for example, I could eat lasagna due to the flatness of the noodle allowing me to control where it went in my mouth but had to avoid spaghetti as the different fine noodles would fall onto the right side of my tongue and mouth where I had no feeling and I would lose track of them and choke. I never looked at food the same way again. Everything was texture, ease of breaking it down, moisture content and spiciness. Too much spice and my graft would get irritated, quickly ending any chance of swallowing anything in that meal. As humans we have an amazing array of foods to choose from out there in the world. I have come to appreciate them all and the little things that make them unique. I have ventured into worlds of food I would never thought possible in the past but now these same foods are among my favorites.

Chapter 26

Working on a Forest Fire

Another, in a long list of things I probably shouldn't have done. It is so hard to let go of what defines you, or at the very least, what you think defines you as a person. Many people think the career makes the man but they are missing the boat. I was one of those people to some extent, but realize now that I was very wrong.

I love fighting forest fires and I think I am pretty good at it. Over the past twenty years I have climbed the ranks of this honorable profession and now get dispatched to some very complex high caliber incidents. After spending a year fighting and recovering from life changing Cancer therapy and then slowly building my strength up while working full time at my old job however, this was not my best choice of activities to participate in.

First of all a side effect of my treatment was an extreme sensitivity to smoke as it badly irritates the graft in the back of my throat. Secondly, sleeping in an abandoned gravel pit on a thin mat for two weeks in the outdoor elements was probably not a good way to stay rested and continue to recover. Than working twelve to fourteen hour days, plus trying to fuel my body with three hours of chewing and 3000 calories was an uphill battle for the entire fire tour.

At the start of the tour, I tipped the scales at 168 lbs. My position kept me out of the smoke for the most part as more of a forecaster and observer of what the fire could and would do. I managed my time well and by the end of the two week tour I had hung onto my weight for the most part. The bad thing was that I was completely exhausted and would need a few days off to recover. Much of my time off was spent horizontal sleeping or on the couch drifting in and out of consciousness as I watched television.

Chapter 27

Caleb's Grad

The graduation of my first born was something I will never forget. As a father this ranks up with the proudest moments in my life. After surviving all that had been thrown my way, this event was overwhelming with emotion. I felt so lucky to be able to just sit there and take in this moment of my child's life. Wave after wave of emotion hit me. I spent the entire proceeding of the diploma presentation crying, then gaining control, then crying again. I couldn't stop the tears flowing. I was a blubbering fool. So much so that my son avoided me as he didn't want his friends seeing me this way. There I sat in the arena after the presentation staring at the floor tears flowing. They just wouldn't stop, I was truly shaken. I didn't want anyone to see me this way. I cried and cried until the last few souls in the arena departed. Then and only then, I looked up and around to be certain no one would be there to witness this display. I gathered myself and after a few minutes headed out to the parking lot to see everyone. I encountered moments of losing myself in the tears again but managed to hang on.

That said, I wouldn't change a thing because I recognized my mortality and just how lucky I truly was. Most people that went through what I had just done did not survive to enjoy a moment like this. I cannot drive this home strongly enough, it is a miracle that I am here today. I find that my emotions are hard to control now, at times when I become overwhelmed with happiness, love, or sadness the tears flow freely. It's scary in a way, as all my life I had learned to hide my feelings and put on a strong face. Now I have lost that ability and my emotions flow free, unchecked. The weeks to come would highlight just how lucky I truly was to be there. The long drive north, back to work, gave me time to think of how I wanted to ensure I did not take anything or any moment in life for granted ever again.

Chapter 28

Strep "A" Blood Borne

The graduation ceremony was draining to say the least and the 600 km drive home after, and back to work compounded that fact. I welcomed the approaching Canada Day long weekend as one to put the feet up and recharge. It was a quiet weekend and Saturday night I was invited to go sit around the fire at the bunkhouse and enjoy a couple of cool ones. I welcomed this opportunity and had a great time reminiscing and being in the company of others. I left relatively early, satisfied and feeling good.

The next morning I awoke with a sore throat. It felt raw and I didn't feel well at all. It was getting harder and harder to shift the thick ropey saliva in my throat as the day went on. After a drink to wash it down everything started to plug up my airway. It felt as if I was choking on my own throat and it was getting progressively harder to breathe. I started to wheeze and struggle for a breath. At this moment I realized I couldn't do this on my own and started to look for help from my landlord whom I was renting a room from. They were outside with company, I yelled with all my might, I was scared now and my feeble voice didn't carry far. Luckily someone had popped into the house for a moment and heard my cry. She came to my assistance and asked if I wanted an ambulance. I said yes, and she hit her husband's Lifeline button. The operator came on and talked to me continuously as I waited for the ambulance. I couldn't talk and was having great difficulty breathing. I was panicking now and my heart was racing at an uncontrollable rate, I was afraid to die. Between the operator and my landlord I had all I could ask for. The landlord happened to have oxygen so they put it on me and I felt some relief as my throat relaxed and I calmed slowly.

The paramedics arrived with the fire department and one reached for my left arm to check my radial pulse. This calmed me further as he was having problems finding a beat. I almost had to laugh, as this was the arm that the graft was taken from. Funny how that is when you can laugh at these times, but knowing that I didn't have an artery to provide a pulse gave some comedy relief to the moment. This further calmed me and I was feeling some relief as I could feel air entering my lungs without a fight. Loaded into the ambulance feeling stabilized I went over my medical history with the paramedic as well as I could. Off we went. On the way we encountered a vehicle accident on the highway and the ambulance stopped to check if there were any injuries before carrying on. Finally we arrived at the hospital and I received a bed in emergency for observation. All seemed well, I did not understand what had just happened to me but I did feel that the worst was behind me.

The nurse told me they would keep me overnight to ensure all was well before sending me home. My landlord had followed me to the hospital and said he would come and get me when I was released. The nurse had given me some sponge swabs to clear the mucus in my throat, it seemed to work well. I started feeling a bit relaxed now and just got comfortable for the night. Later on a nurse stopped by and asked if I was thirsty. I said I was and she gave me a glass of water with a small straw in it so I could take tiny sips to moisten my mouth from time to time.

The result of my first drink, after she left, was the moisture reacting with the thick saliva in my throat and making it like glue. My already challenged and inflamed airway was in trouble again. I hit the panic button again and started to struggle as I choked, saying I couldn't breathe. The nurses rushed over and a Doctor came up. All I remember was feeling like I was losing the battle again and going to die. During my gasps for air saying I can't breathe, I was looking at the doctor on call that night saying "He can breathe" and blowing me off like I was just being over dramatic. The anger filled me and I wanted to do nothing more but make sure that Doctor came with me. If I wasn't going to make it, he was coming along for the ride. They say fight or flight comes at these times and I was ready to fight. It took a number of orderlies, nurses and such to keep me pinned down until the meds took effect paralyzing me. I can remember voices and hearing what was going on but I couldn't open my eyes or move. I willed my eyes to open but nothing.

When I woke next I found myself intubated in the Intensive Care Unit (ICU). Intubated means they have shoved a plastic tube down your throat to allow air to flow into your lungs before your airway closes and breath is not possible. Once it closes it is not easy if at all possible to do. It's a good thing that emerge Doctor figured out I couldn't breathe eventually and had half of a clue what to do because I was very lucky to survive a life threatening event yet again. I don't know whether to punch him for almost killing me or hug him for saving my life. I guess he is only human after all and should be allowed a mistake once in a while.

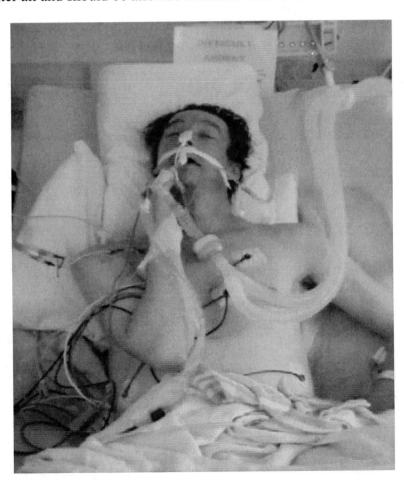

The nurses were very good to me, putting eye drops in to keep my eyes from drying out and in general just taking care of me. One asked if there was anyone they could call. I couldn't talk but was used to writing to replace my voice and wrote them that I wanted to see my kids. This hurt a great deal but I just didn't think I was going to make it and couldn't go without telling my kids I love them. The call got through and they started the 600 km drive to see their Dad in hospital. I can't imagine their thoughts at this time but I didn't know what else to do. I had to see them if only one more time. I arranged with friends to get them set up in a hotel room and waited for their arrival. Sixty minutes after the kids arrived I got the news I was being transferred and flying to Edmonton. The X-rays they had taken had shown a shadow in my throat that they took to be the return of cancer in the form of another tumor. This was something beyond their abilities so they chose to send me back to where it all began, to the University of Alberta Hospital in Edmonton.

I was scared and felt bad for putting my kids through that long journey of wondering. It was good to see them but, I would have to say goodbye, if only for a short while. Off I went, loaded into an ambulance and off to the airport. They loaded me into a small plane which had just enough room for my paramedics and my stretcher. Arriving in Edmonton I was loaded into another ambulance and off to my new digs. Of note, was that I had no clothes. You see I was in a housecoat and boxers when this whole thing started. I had nothing. It seems one can never be ready for such an emergency, things just happen and we have to deal with them as they come.

Back to the ICU in Edmonton I went. Not sure how long I was in there, but during my stay I managed to participate in a research project related to taking a certain drug in order to improve survival chances in ICU. My bed was easy to spot it was the one with the big difficult airway sign above it. I continued to survive and was transferred to my old ward on the third floor. This time I got my own room where I was quarantined as Strep "A" Blood Borne was the source of all my misery.

A contagious disease, Strep Throat for most can be a nuisance and aggravation with a sore throat, fever, or swollen lymph nodes occurring for a few days, before recovery. For a recovering cancer patient with a weakened immune system and open wound on his chin providing a nice entry point from an ongoing infection this can be a fatal occurrence. A variety of strep throat is Strep "A" blood borne meaning being in the blood. The bacteria can then enter into the bloodstream and work itself throughout your body affecting various favorite organs perhaps and complicating an already troubled throat and airway leading to your demise. My throat remained inflamed for about 4 to 6 months after my initial hospitalization as a result of this infection.

Again I am not sure when the tube was removed from my throat and replaced by a trache but I guess I proved that doctor wrong in Fort McMurray after all, I really couldn't breathe. Not really an argument I want to be on the winning side of too often. At least he was better at his job putting the tube in then his bed side manner would suggest. I owe him my life so I guess I can cut him some slack. My specialist was amazed at the work they had done in order to get me intubated as my throat was almost swollen shut. He reaffirmed the prognosis that I was again, lucky to be here.

A new trache installed, it was back to the work of recovery. Starting all over again from scratch for a second time, I did not look forward to the battle ahead of swallowing. I knew the work that was ahead of me and just how much it would suck. But what choice did I have, I wasn't going to eat meals through a straw for the rest of my sorry life, I loved food and enjoying what food has to offer. It's more than just nutrition. It is a social medium in which to live life to the fullest. How many of you understand the mechanics of a swallow? It is something that I never gave a thought to until I couldn't do it. As babies we come into this world and immediately look to suckle on a mother's breast, swallowing and crying or using our voices is what we do from that first instant of life in the world. It is how we survive and communicate, instinctively. From that moment on we are eating and talking machines without a thought about it. It is amazing what is all involved in the swallowing of different foods. Regardless of the challenge I was willing to do what it took to live again.

Back to Ward 3 at the University Hospital for a second stay this time I received my own room. It has its benefits being immune deficient and perhaps contagious. Most of the wards nurses from my first visit were still there and not very happy to see me. The only way they wanted to see me again was perhaps bearing donuts or other baked goods on a social stop over. Not by any means, bed ridden with a new trache and not enough strength to help myself. I do recommend their care though as it is second to none.

It seems to be a repeating theme but without their help and many others like them I had no chance of making it to today and writing these words for you. There will always be a special place in my heart for the many nurses of Ward 3. My respect for them is unmatched. They took care of me and nurtured me back to health.

A credit to the youth of today was one young man who had volunteered his summer in 2009 to spend time learning about what they do in a hospital, and helping out the nurses of ward 3 wherever he could. He couldn't have been much older than 16. He spent hours I am sure, just visiting the patients throughout the ward and trying to make them more comfortable, chatting, and sometimes getting them a small snack or drink at times. Once I could speak again, he used to check on me quite often and listen to my stories of firefighting, cancer fighting and life in general or he would just sit quietly as I cried sometimes. My voice was weak and sometimes I was too depressed or exhausted to speak, but he always came by. I have mixed feelings about him being there. It was great to have such an experience available to him to learn from, but at the same time some of the subject matter and situations encountered, force someone his age such as my own children to grow up faster than they have to, and I don't know if I like that very much.

Chapter 29

My Second PEG Tube

Being familiar with the challenges ahead and knowing how high a hill I had to climb, I reached out for a helping hand in the form of PEG tube number two and my third belly button. This idea however, inspired a great debate with my specialists head intern, who was in charge of my care during his absence. One thing surgeons and doctors don't like to do is cut into you if they don't have to. No matter how minor the surgery is perceived to be, it is still surgery and things can go very wrong. That said, one must weigh the risks with the benefits and judge as to which is greater in order to make a fully informed decision.

I had a distinct advantage in this debate though. I had been down this road before, and I knew what I was facing. I knew the value of the PEG tube and that it could help me ride out the bad days. Some days nausea, fatigue or depression would make it hard to put in the effort to eat the old fashion way. Without the PEG tube I would lose ground on these days and have to work all the harder the next. One step forward and two steps back without the tube, but with the tube I could ride out these days and still maintain the full amount of calories needed to sustain me and help me gain back the weight I lost again. I think I slipped down to the 155 pounds area during my hospital stay this time and couldn't afford to lose anymore.

Back and forth we debated my request, me on paper, the intern with his voice. He finally gave in to my badgering. Every time he walked in my door I asked him for it and I am glad for that because had I not received the PEG I know for certain I would have been booking an extended stay at the hospital again. I think his main concern was first the risks associated with surgery and secondly that I would be lazy and rely on the tube too much to feed me prolonging my recovery.

I understood his concerns but I also knew the work involved and told him straight up that this was something I needed to get over the hump. I promised that I would do the work required of me. Now you must realize that for me to eat something like two scrambled eggs with a little bit of cheese melted in it, I was looking at a good 2o minutes and a large glass or two of juice to wash it down. A small plate of food would take about 1.5 liters of liquid and a good solid hour of chewing to finish it off.

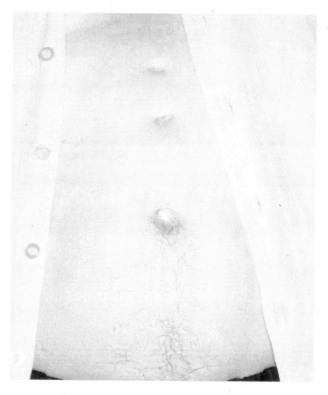

My requirement was 3000 calories a day again, in order to gain one pound a week. I spent two hours attached to the tube feed and two hours chewing for the first few weeks. Slowly I gained weight and strength. I started taking more calories by mouth then by PEG tube. About an hour and a half on the PEG feed then close to three hours chewing every day. Time yourself next meal and you will find most meals you finish eating in 15 minutes or less. Imagine sitting at the table for an hour just chewing one little bite at a time then swallowing it with a drink washing it down every time. Your food starts to get cold but you don't care because reheating it half a dozen times before your done is just a pointless waste of time. That time could be spent chewing so you may finally leave the table sustained for a few hours before its time to eat again.

As I mentioned earlier there is more to swallowing then you think. Many people that have gone through my treatment regime cannot eat half of the things I do or did. One thing I must say is that I tried anything and everything to find out if it went down easy and now know every trick in the book to pound on calories. I started with foods like eggs, yogurt, and cream soups heavy in calories and super shakes of my own recipe. I could put together a 2500 calorie shake that was nutritional in about five minutes. Ice cream, yogurt, milk, banana, loads of frozen fruits, peanut butter, nutella, you name it I put it in there. No diet stuff allowed. The secret to gaining weight was eat high calorie healthy foods but make it as little work as possible to allow for success. If you eat eggs, you mix them with milk, cook them in butter and melt cheese in them and have them with ketchup to boost the calories in your meal without adding more bites. Drink juices and milk instead of water. Homogenized milk has more calories than skim milk. Chocolate milk is just as good if you are like me and don't care for drinking normal milk.

For swallowing different foods and drinks there are different challenges. Did you know that water is the hardest liquid to swallow and milk is one of the easiest? Liquids have various textures and consistency that make them harder or easier to swallow. Water is the thinnest liquid and tea and coffee are noticeably easier to get down.

With meats and fish the finer the grain the easier the swallow. Fish is a soft consistency which is easy to break up and has a moisture content that assists in the swallow. I rate fish and meats as follows from easiest to hardest in swallowing:

1) Fish
2) Deli Meats of uniform consistency, no mustard seeds or peppercorns etc.
3) Ham
4) Pork Ribs (Baby Back)

5)   Dark meat chicken and turkey (It is moister)

6)   White Meat chicken and turkey

7)   Pork Chops and tenderloin

8)   Ground Beef

9)   Beef steak

So there I was winning the battle, getting stronger by the day and then the scares started coming in with the dreaded H1N1 all over the news. I had never been for a flu shot in my life but I was thinking I had better get one now.

I looked up the information on where to get a shot and headed out. The line ups were huge everywhere and I was too weak to sit there all day so I went home and thought I would wait out the rush. Next thing I knew there was a shortage on the vaccine, the demand was extremely high and so they started to prioritize who could get a shot. I didn't make the category so there I sat waiting for my turn. It was about this time that my favorite hockey team, the Calgary Flames, wait for it, NOT, made the news. It seems they managed to jump the line and get access to the vaccine somehow. Connections, connections hmm, makes one think a little doesn't it. So, let's get back to my point. I never did receive a vaccine because while I was waiting I came across a flu bug which I can only guess to be H1N1. I could barely lift my body vertical for about three weeks. It was all I could do just to pour a few cans in my PEG tube feed bag and get some nutrition, going to the bathroom took serious planning, thought and conviction. The thought of depends undergarments did cross my mind on more than one occasion, where I just couldn't drag myself along.

So if I did have H1N1, you must be wondering, why I didn't just go to the hospital. Well, I have an answer for you and that is, if I went back in, I didn't know if I could ever get out of it again. You see a hospital setting wears on your mindset and strength. It can be depressing after a while. The nurses are fantastic, but it still doesn't change the sterile environment that you are living in. It is not a comfortable place to be. On top of that, the place was already full of flu victims and the last thing I needed was another complication of some disease or superbug. Good thing I had my

PEG tube back up for needed nutrition because it wouldn't have been my choice to stay at home if I hadn't had it. I couldn't eat and a slow starvation would have ensued on me for sure. If only that head intern could have seen me then, saying I told you so, admit it. I was right, you were wrong. I cheated death again.

Chapter 30

Depression

Depression is a reality. That said, after what I have been through, if I wasn't depressed off and on at some time or another I think that would worry me more. I find this topic very difficult to write about because for the past few months I have been flowing in and out of a depression in waves. The weight of the world just becomes too great and you can't hold it up anymore. Sometimes I just hurt, every needle, every pain of every step, every time I tried to swallow and started to choke, sometimes I try to say a simple hello to someone I have known for years but the name escapes me and I become frustrated and want to go curl up in a corner and hide. Although the doctors did a fantastic job, and many who look at me don't see the scars, I look in the mirror and all I can see is the damage and disfigurement left behind, the scars magnify themselves on my neck and chin. Down days happen, and we just hope they pass sooner than later.

All I know is that sometimes I fall into a dark place and with each passing moment it gets harder and harder to climb out of it. I just want to give up fighting and let it all end. The big thing here is that there is a difference from wanting to die to stop the pain and being suicidal. One scenario no matter how unlikely it seems at the time; shows that hope and optimism will eventually raise its head again and bring back that smile which everyone, hopes to see. The other scenario shows pain and despair and no way out, an utter helplessness. Anger comes easy, frustration, anxiety and the why me cries return. At times you are sitting there, perhaps in your office and you are thankful you have a door you can close because you have started to cry for no reason in particular other than a sad thought entering your mind.

At these times you need the support of a loved one and some professional help. Most large companies have health programs you can access through your work. The Cross Cancer Institute also has some help for you there and your Doctor is always there to help you along. Reach out, talk to someone and get the help you need early.

I did a great job of being strong and working my butt off to physically get back to work and what I thought was life. Funny how I preach that 90 percent of surviving Cancer is in your mind as the body can recover from anything and will bounce back. I just raced back to work at the first moment I thought my body could handle it, and forgot to take time to heal my mind. Take the time and heal your mind, you just went through multiple traumas and death scares and need time to reflect and deal with the mental aspects of it before you can function well in your life and work. Nothing will ever be the same again, learn from my mistake and use the time you are given to heal both mind and body.

Chapter 31

Christmas Again

The third Christmas since my initial surgery was supposed to be a good one. I had been working hard, on eating and was looking for results. I couldn't wait to get to my sisters and fill up a plate of turkey and all the fixings. I was going to enjoy this one. I didn't care if I had to sit there all day and chew, I had decided I was going to mound my plate high and enjoy every morsel. The previous year it had taken over three hours to eat a small plate. This year would be different as I had been working on my swallow technique with much improvement in efficiency. I wasn't as scared to choke on things and had a better understanding of how to systematically attack my meal.

Happy times were here again or so I thought. Then the message came down. One of my good friends had ended up in hospital again with heart issues. Since it was near where I was going for dinner and I was making the trip into Edmonton anyway, I decided to visit. I just sucked it up, as the last place I wanted to be again was in a hospital at this time of year. I really don't like going but I make myself go as I know what it means to get a visit from a friend when you are trapped in there for long periods over and over again.

A mind can only take so much without the support of others to prop you up or tell you it's going to be ok. Some days you just want it to be over, and plead to whoever will listen to that inside voice, to just end the misery. You look forward, but see nothing but pain and wonder how you will go on. It is so hard the path ahead and you feel so tired of the fight. That is a little taste of what my friend and I have in common, so I knew to drag my butt in there and do what I could even if it be nothing but be a sound board for support. The visit weighed on my mind but I left thinking I had been of some comfort and maybe a little bit of help to him.

It was time to lighten up the mood and go eat a feast of Christmas Dinner. I mounded my plate to its maximum capacity and got comfortable. Slowly those around me got up and left the table to do the dishes, play a few games, or simply just relax and loosen the waist band. I ate and ate, emptying out trays and pots of food before they were hauled away to be stowed for leftovers and cleaned up. Two hours later I sat there full as can be with a wide satisfied grin on my face. I had eaten two mounded plates of food in what I considered record time. My jaw was sore from grinding up all that chow but I didn't care, I had a good feeling in my tummy. Life felt almost normal again and I already looked forward to next year's feast.

Chapter 32

Wanting to Return to Work

Once the holiday festivities ended my thoughts, which were once again in a positive state of mind, turned to going back to work and getting on with life so I picked up the phone and called the insurance people. Knowing that this would be my second attempt at returning to work they wanted to make sure I was fit to return and requested a letter from my Doctor stating I was alright to go back. I set up an appointment, met the Doctor, and requested a letter of clearance for the end of January. He seemed okay with this. I left the paperwork with him to forward on and waited for the insurance company to get back to me.

The insurance company then hooked me up with an assessor that would provide me some assistance in getting back into shape via a fitness consultant and then setting a slow as you go back to work schedule. At first I was bitter, as I just wanted to get back to normal life but then it sunk in and I realized just how far off I was from being physically able to handle any semblance of work.

My first visit to the gym left me exhausted after two minutes speed walking on the treadmill. Weight training had me struggling with small weights that I am sure a slight ten year old child would have no problem lifting. The cool down walk around the track is where I shined just before I hit the locker room. The work ahead of me was a big hill to climb and I left the gym tired yet satisfied and feeling positive. My doctor had made the right call, no doubt my mind could have dragged my butt through work and eventually it would have gotten easier as time went on, but I would have been walking a tight rope the whole time and most likely regressed in my health in short order ending up worse off then I started.

You get out what you put in so I started going to the gym four times a week, sometimes five and working out my entire routine for a good solid hour. Two or three of these times a week found me working with my fitness trainer after speech therapy. I was going hard and seeing the progress on both fronts. My voice got stronger as my body built muscle. After a month I could actually see something resembling a bicep again forming on my arm. My skeletal frame once again had muscle encasing it.

My energy level increased, I ate more foods with confidence, I felt stronger, and was ready to start the graduated daily hours schedule to get back at work full time. I continued to work out, eat healthy, feel positive, and started with a few hours three days a week slowly building to a full schedule again. My attitude was great and I was smiling again everywhere I went.

My boss was understanding and helped me integrate into work slowly. First, I started with project work. Then I slowly took over my operational program and the responsibilities which go with it. I didn't feel overwhelmed, and my positive energy flowed. Being positive and being around positive people was very important to me at this time. I was very happy but what I didn't know was that this happiness was very fragile and any negativity would be accentuated and drag me down. Within a couple months there, I was back in the routine of work and life.

Chapter 33

PET Scan

A day of truth is what results from the PET scan. Bad news or good news is not differentiated here. It is just a matter of fact type thing. Is the Cancer present or not, period. This can be a difficult time for many, but a bit freeing for others regardless of the news given. I guess the gist of it is, if you are lit up like a roman candle, it isn't a good thing. This is because the radioactive material they inject you with, binds with the cancer cells and lights them up so they are very visible.

The machine that conducts the scan is like two big donuts, with you in the middle, spinning around you taking pictures from every angle possible I guess, searching out that telltale glow of Cancer.

Prior to being placed in the machine was very relaxing. I remember having to sit in a comfy lazy boy type chair very still with my feet up for about an hour. This was after receiving a very quick IV of some radioactive liquid that only filled a little under a centimeter of IV line. The IV was over before it started or so it seemed. I guess the purpose of sitting so still is to allow the radioactive material to spread slowly and evenly through your entire body. No fire works for me that day, as I was lucky and no Cancer was detected this time.

I think it was around this time that it dawned on me to ask my radiation specialist so when will I be considered cancer free. The response was never, it is just that the more years out you get past five without it coming back, the less likely the chance you will have it show up again. I find that concept hard to swallow because I am not terminal as far as I understand the definition to be, but yet I am not cured either. I am just out there floating in between somewhere.

Chapter 34

Speech Therapy

The days I went to work out with the trainer, I also went in and took my speech therapy. My voice had become a whisper without any power and I struggled to enunciate anything clearly enough to be understood or heard for that matter, in a loud setting such as a cafeteria or shopping mall food court.

Now, no matter how funny it seems singing notes high and low to the sound of Ahhhhhhhh you must do the work that is asked of you. This goes for any aspect of your treatment. The reason for this is that they know best how to get a result from the exercise you are doing. No matter how strange things seem to you, get over it and do it. The techniques have been proven or you would not be doing them outside of a research setting.

It felt strange driving in my car or sitting in my bedroom in the basement doing my voice exercises when my kids came home from school with friends and such. But, that said, it reaped rewards. Upon my arrival back at work I completed a 45 minute presentation to a group of over 50 people in an auditorium successfully and can only thank my therapist for that result. I have had to learn to talk from scratch twice in the past four years and without speech therapy a hoarse whisper is all that would have remained of my voice.

Having a voice that can be heard gives you a confidence. Having to sit in a corner and only be able to whisper something to someone in a quiet setting is a recipe for withdrawal into one's self and in my case the onset of a serious depression. Downward spiral and no desire for life would have ensued, so I am very thankful indeed for the help I have received.

Chapter 35

My 3 Belly Button's Article

(the title worked there so I thought why not here)

One day at speech therapy I was asked if I would like to perhaps write an article for a newsletter at IRSM. IRSM is the Institute for Reconstructive Sciences in Medicine, located within the Misericordia Hospital in Edmonton, Alberta. Their role in my therapy is a combination of monitoring my swallow progress and assisting me with ways to make it more efficient which they did, providing speech therapy for both clarity and volume, and then tracking the health of my teeth which are slowly degrading due to lack of blood flow caused by the radiation I took in my jaw area. Eventually my teeth will most likely start to rot out from the roots and begin to breakdown. I will then need a full surgical removal of them and then posts implanted to attach a set of permanently reconstructed dentures one day hopefully not too soon. Helping with the simple things in life that one takes for granted until they no longer have the ability to do them, is the basis of how they helped me.

The newsletter is for patients going through similar things and the health professionals whose business is helping those same individuals. Articles and information are submitted by all. I found this process therapeutic and helpful in my own healing as an outlet, and once I started to put words down, it did not take long to get it done and submitted.

The reason it was called, my three belly buttons is simple, I now have three belly buttons or so I call them, running up the middle of my abdomen. One caused at birth, one with my first PEG Tube as described earlier and a third created by my second PEG Tube. It is interesting looking back, at the various stages of what got me here where I am today. I have learned so much, and some of these things have helped others so I have in a small way already accomplished what I set out to do. There is nothing more satisfying then receiving feedback from a friend or stranger alike, saying that they took my article to a loved one and they took strength to deal with their own situation and comfort in mind from it. I feel honored in some twisted way of fate, to be in a position to help those who are at their most vulnerable.

Chapter 36

Bone Infection in Jaw

All things considered, I think I have had an easy ride compared to what could have been. I was lucky to have only minor complications from surgery, and that I was strong of mind and able to fight. Funny how life is, as I had gained about 30 pounds, six months before finding out I had cancer and that extra weight may have been my saving grace.

The only complication I had after initial treatment that needed further attention was a bone infection in my jaw related to the metal plate that was installed to hold my jaw in place as the bone healed and welded itself back together. This occurrence is not out of the ordinary as some people's bodies just reject the plate. That said though, the bone still has to heal together prior to removal of the plate. So after surgery a year and a half passed by with me having an open sore on the bottom of my chin that would puss and scab over, then break, drain, and start all over again repeating the scenario over and over again.

A couple of days after I was hospitalized with the Strep "A" I was to see my specialist to discuss the removal of the plate and a final end to the routine cycle of this infection. You become a bit self-conscious with an open sore always on your chin, never knowing when it will decide to start draining.

As you have probably guessed by now, having my life threatened by another infection in the form of Strep "A" took priority so I missed my appointment and would have to wait until I recovered from this new scenario before worrying about this minor irritation to my life.

Eventually this happened and 2.5 years after the initial surgery to remove my tumor, I was scheduled again to go under the knife and get the plate on my chin removed. The bone was long healed together and I was on the road to recovery.

Step one was remove the plate, step two, take care of the infection. Within 24 hours of taking step one, I was feeling good and had got back to my after appointment routine of hitting up my favorite fish and chips place at the mall. I remember it well, I looked like I had been mugged and had my chin smacked by a busted beer bottle. The girl and guy behind the counter couldn't resist asking what had happened so I told them with a smile of sorts on my face. Every time I visit that establishment after an Edmonton appointment the young woman still working there acknowledges me remembering that day and says hi. It is something that I have always appreciated and has lifted my spirits on more than one occasion. Once published, I think I will drop a copy off for her and let her see how she does have a great impact in the lives of people she serves.

The first step completed, it was on to phase two, taking care of the infection and time for a PICC line installation. A PICC line is like a heavy duty IV line that is almost a permanent installation in your arm and used for continual long term intravenous drug therapy. I had mine for six weeks.

I got lucky again as my therapy was only once a day at the same time every day, whereas on the weekends I would go into emerge and week days into a clinic. I had a bit of traveling that I had to complete during this time so my Doctor would send orders identifying dates I would be in a particular town so that the various hospitals could ensure they had the appropriate medications available for me. I must say, the system did itself proud and I had no interruption in the regime required. Some not so lucky would have to go three times a day at the same time every day. I cannot imagine how exhausted I would have been after that. Up all hours of the night waiting for my meds in the Emergency Department. Heavy dose antibiotics knock you down as it is, and that would have laid me out for the whole six week term. I would not have being able to function as a normal human being just climbing in and out of bed to eat something get your meds and then go back home to lie down would have been my maximum.

Chapter 37

Finding Happiness

Despite the past few years were filled with separation of marriage, trying to still maintain a close relationship with my children 600 km away, and a fight for my life on more than one occasion. I was in a good place in my life at this juncture you might say. I actually thought about socializing again, taking a class in something like cooking or writing. Just hoping to maybe meet some people, maybe even meet a nice lady I could go on a date with. I wanted to have more in my life then work and my children. I wanted some selfish little bit of happiness just for me. Call it, my me time.

I never thought I would find someone again. I wasn't looking, and even went as far as to say on the few dates I had, that I wasn't looking for anything resembling commitment or seriousness. I just wanted to meet some people and have some adult conversation that wasn't related to work, family or cancer and escape for a few hours into a world without stress. Funny how when you are not looking for something, it just appears. There it is before you, waiting for you to grab hold of it. Her name is Jeanette and she is that something I wasn't looking for, that pleasant surprise in life.

You are allowed to be happy. No matter how many times you think, I must have done something really bad in order to get Cancer like somehow you control the fates. You really don't, and really are allowed to be happy again, so reach out and take that chance when it stands in front of you. I did and without it sometimes I wonder if I would have made it this far. Don't under estimate the power of those that love you in your recovery. A positive aura in the air is a powerful thing. It is one that can move mountains and make the impossible seem possible again. It allows dreams to form where only nightmares existed and brings back the will to go on, tenfold. I found such an opportunity before me in the form of an honest, open, loving woman and I embraced it. I admit I was scared initially. Not wanting anyone too close to me because what if the Cancer came back, I didn't want to be a burden on another life. I was very open about my cancer from day one with her. One day she mentioned that she had been thinking about us and the cancer thing. She had come up with the thought that tomorrow one of us could get hit by a bus as we walked across the street or get in an accident any number of ways. Neither of us could tell the future, so maybe it was okay to take a chance on each other. I don't feel guilty for this little selfish act of wanting and now finding happiness, and I don't think anyone should. You deserve some happiness in life, you just lived through hell and back and it is time you enjoyed a little heaven on earth, so do it. It is a time to live life for the precious gift it is.

Chapter 38

Video Interview

Sometimes you get asked to give something back after the second, third, and fourth chances you have been given. To help others with your case or your story is a gift bestowed on you by your survival to date. Take a moment from your day and do something to help someone when asked. When you see a void that needs to be filled, fill it. Could it be so simple you ask? The answer is simply put, yes it can.

My speech therapist asked me one day if I would be willing to do a video interview, for her to present to a large group of speech and swallow therapist students, at the University of Alberta. I responded yes, that would be no problem, and got her to send me a list of questions so I could prepare myself for the interview.

The basis of the interview is that she wanted to give the students an understanding of what we as Cancer patients go through. Starting from day one, when we find out we have Cancer, until present day and all the struggles, victories and challenges we face in between. She had written a short list of questions and we set up the date.

The date approached and Jeanette offered to go with me for support. We took a couple days off work so we could head into the city five hours away and make me a movie star. Nerves of the unknown set in, introductions were done and off to the little interview room we went. The camera was set up and zoomed in on my face for the big close-up shot that would last the whole session. Jeanette held my hand as Gabi asked the question, "How did it feel when you were told that you had cancer?" Off I went starting from day one and just puking it all up, not stopping for about 45 minutes. It was a rollercoaster of emotions, some more painful than others, some happy or funny times, some silent holes filled with tears and sadness. I looked up and Gabi looked at the questions list, depleted and most of them answered to some degree at this point and asked what advice I could give to the caregivers. Off I went again for about a half hour this time. It was easy to go on and on because I had so much to say that I wanted to cram into what seemed like 5 minutes.

You see these care providers see you for a baseline assessment at the beginning before any physical trauma occurs. Then again they see you after you are recovered, to sort of finish you off giving you some tools to lead a normal life with. They don't comprehend the value of what they do for you the patient, so sometimes they need to be told and shown. I guess my video was a success with not a dry eye in the house, and many not to forget the importance of what they do, too soon.

Chapter 39

Cavities Cavities

A side effect of radiation at the dental level when it is applied to the mouth and throat area is lack of blood flow to the teeth and destruction of saliva glands. Both of these items are important to a healthy smile as they help provide invaluable nutrients and cleanliness to it.

Effects of treatment are continually ongoing and creep up on you as the days go by. One day I went to the dentist and wham, the word came down, I had eleven cavities and had to schedule two visits to get them looked after. This was a sign of things to come. The first appointment took care of the right side of my face and seven cavities. You can imagine how frozen my face was, numb right up to the eyeball socket. I left there with absolutely no feeling and unaware that I had bit my tongue and lip to the point of bleeding on my way down to the LRT subway train. I look back and now understand why people were looking strangely at me that day. Face lop sided and puffy with blood running down my chin and a stupid smile on my face heading to my swallow therapist appointment that I would not be able to function much at due to my lack of feeling.

My new reality is that I am lucky to be in this situation. The majority of patients treated as I was, do not have teeth anymore. If I heard correctly at my last appointment, there is actually only one other person in this province that still has his teeth. So although my teeth are slowly chipping away at the roots, they are still there and they are still real so I can keep on smiling for a while yet. Speaking of chipping, I am not sure if it was piece of tooth or a piece of filling, but a chunk broke off while chewing a bit of celery at a retirement luncheon today. Little losses and big victories is all I can hope for and continue to work towards.

One day my teeth will be beyond all help possible. Then they will start snapping in half with brittleness, and it will be time for complete surgical removal and the implanting of posts as anchors for a new set of choppers. The line ups are long for that procedure and can be over a year in the waiting so here is hoping that that reality is years off. I can only dream that I remain the special exception to the rule, for a while yet. The side effects from radiation are definitely an ongoing concern, but oh well just continue to smile and life will go on.

Chapter 40

Divorce

Finalizing a relationship such as marriage is a traumatic and wearing event in anyone's life. When you are healthy, it can really weigh on you. It can be very nasty at times, and there is just no good thing about it pretty much on any front. It is just something that has to be done to allow life to move on in a happy healthy direction. When you are recovering from a disease such as Cancer, these events can affect your physical health as well as your mental health. Any large stressor in life may adversely affect you.

Your physical well-being may be compromised and you should seek the advice of a health professional as soon as possible when you are starting to feel sick or overwhelmed. Any event that may trigger a high emotional response such as a traumatic accident to a loved one, death of a loved one, someone close to you being diagnosed with cancer or anything along those lines has the potential of long lasting adverse reactions for your fragile shell and should be addressed once recognized. Little problems don't go away, they just pile up until they all fall off the shelf at the same time and you become lost and in need of some serious help.

My present situation is like two sides of a coin. On one side I have love, support and sanity and on the other side I have stress, turmoil, and for a while an unhealthy situation that threatened to bring my world down. I have learned something over the past few years and put in a call for help which has being answered, and is slowly helping me pull it back together again.

Chapter 41

Counseling

The body is resilient and will rebuild if provided the proper building blocks such as diet and the gradual building of intensity in exercise. The mind however, is a little more fragile you might say. You cannot see all that is hurt or wrong in the mind, as it stores those things away in order to protect you. It does not forget however, no matter what you think, all it has done is hidden those bad times and painful memories in a dark corner somewhere. It needs time to heal and counseling is a great help in this direction.

It has been close to four years now since my diagnosis with Cancer, and I am once again facing a long term disability situation being unable to function at work. Life and the stress that comes with it have caught up with me. Without counseling I don't think I would be here today typing out my story. I looked to counseling when life and work started to overwhelm me, but I think I went too late. I had hit the point of no return and was slipping over the edge. I hid it well from those close to me and put on a strong face. Meanwhile I started going to counseling sessions as much as once a week. Stressors started to weigh on me. Things like commencing mutually agreeable divorce proceedings that appeared as if they would be amicable blew up in my face. Constant trips to the doctor and for work, off I went, 450 kms down a snow covered icy highway that seems to claim a life every week. I had ongoing problems with infection and boils resulting in multi antibiotic treatments. These wiped out my immune system, and laid me out horizontal with an exhaustion that compounded daily and never seemed to end. I was running on empty. I was served with court papers for divorce and that appeared to be the final straw that broke my mind. I went for a session, walked in the door, and after seeing the look on my face, the next moments were spent assessing me doing tests for depression and suicide then telling me I have to go see my doctor and take medical leave from work. Words such as hypertension, a heart attack waiting to happen and death were the topic of the day.

It probably didn't help that I had used all my sick days up prior to this event and was now using all my annual leave up for doctor's appointments. I was so worried about getting sick that I got sick. I had deep depression, scored in the extreme range and high anxiety. I was easy to anger and ready to snap at any moment. I was getting feelings off and on of pure rage. I just wanted to smash something. Road rage was a given every time I got behind the wheel in this town. More than once, I wanted to slam my gear shift into park, jump out of my seat and start jumping up and down on someone's windshield behind me. I was losing touch with reality and control of my emotions. I could cry at a sad thought and many times had to close my office door to let it out of my system unknown to my peers and gather myself.

I hurt. My girlfriend helped me along, and gave me strength to face the day, but I was broken and in need of fixing. The thing is, unlike a cut, or severed muscle, or tumor, you just can't cut out the bad part and stitch up your mind or put a bandage on it to make it all better. There are drugs to help you feel better but there is a lot of rest and work between feeling better and getting better. My mind throbs with pain at the thought of it all. It has been almost four months and the simple stresses of daily living set me off from time to time but I am working on it.

Chapter 42

Writing this Book

Part of my therapy and a way to healing, was to write it out of me. So day by day I started writing a little bit here, then a little bit there. A story started to form. My story, the one you have been reading today. It was suggested to me in counseling that I have a good story that may help others and that is what I hope to tell. I have a gift given to me from circumstance. I have an opportunity of something good to come out of something that was very hard to deal with in my life. It is my reward to myself in a way, for surviving the turmoil of the past few years battles. I would like nothing more than to make someone's life easier, by learning from my experience, how to avoid or at least prepare one's self, for all the misery they have ahead that may be similar to what I have journeyed through.

Chapter 43

Tax Audit

The two things in life that you can never hide from are death and taxes. The past few years has taught me a valuable lesson in both of these areas but death will hopefully wait a while so let us touch on taxes. Oh where to start. I presently live outside of the community of my main health provider. Although things are improving, and some cancer treatments and therapies are becoming more available in rural Alberta. Most of the therapies, treatments, equipment and specialists can be found in the major urban centers. Not all of us live in these centers so there are expenses associated with travel, meals, basic needs and accommodation that will be incurred in order to obtain this treatment.

This can be a burden of expense that may be hard to take on at the time but the news is not all bad. With some good solid record and receipt keeping practices you can find some relief at the years end when you submit your taxes and deductions. These expenses such as mileage, hotel receipts, meals and such are covered at a km rate for your car, and in the absence of receipts a daily rate for meals and accommodation. Sometimes these bills add up to some very large deduction, say for example $20000. This in turn triggers alarm bells in the tax auditors head, screaming "how can this persons medical expenses be so much", he must be trying to rip off the system. That said, the letter arrives saying you are being audited and they need proof within 30 days so be ready to provide it.

There is something wrong with a system, where the very sick who have enough daily stress to deal with, get audited! How is this going to help them get better so that they may pay more taxes I ask? Some of these Cancer survivors or patients are hanging on the brink of death and feel helpless and weak. There were many days where I could not fight another moment, the hill was just too high to climb and I just wanted to give in and curl up on the floor in a little ball and die. Rather than questioning every appointment they have gone to and asking them to take all their energy they were using on their respective health and refocus it on tax audits, how about making the system a little more user friendly for them. Maybe discuss with respective provinces ideas on record sharing that would provide supporting documentation to the person your auditing's claim so that a burden is removed from the individual who is trying to survive the assault on his or her health.

Here are a few things I learned the hard way and am still learning as I am in the middle of an audit at this moment as follows:

1)   Alberta Health Care can provide you a summary of your health service record for the past year free of charge. Phone them up in January and ask them to send you a copy of the past years appointments and such for tax audit purposes. They will print it off and send it to you.

2)   Maintain a health expense file for each year. I didn't do this until recently. It only took a few years to finally have the strength to start organizing.

3)   Things to include in this file are:

   a)   Yearly Health Care Record

   b)   Cost of health insurance plan, for example Blue Cross

   c)   Receipts from prescriptions, you want to show your portion paid plus not all cancer medications are covered by health plans.

   d)   Parking passes for appointments.

   e)   Receipts from meals on travel.

   f)   Hotel or accommodation receipts.

   g)   Record of Mileage.

   h)   Gas receipts.

   i)   Medical equipment costs.

   j)   Anything related to getting to your appointment and your treatment and therapy should be included.

Just because they say there is a daily rate you can claim in lieu of receipts does not mean they will not ask for this detail when they audit you.

I would like to thank Revenue Canada at this time for the extra stress in my life that I really didn't need, and I wish you the reader all the best, hoping you never require it. After much luck I have survived so far and finally know what to keep on file. Funny how the importance of these items doesn't come to surface until you least need it in your life.

Chapter 44

Feelings of Betrayal of Loyalty to Job

I have worked over 20 years for the same organization and in my health struggles I have a feeling of betrayal that I cannot shake. The road to my health requires a change in location as well as duties. I do not have the capacity left in my tank to fight anymore. I feel beaten and broken. Lately all the stresses of the past few years of battle have caught up to me at once and shook me like a rag doll. I just want to sit and cry sometimes, and painfully admit that I have, on more than one occasion lately.

I reached out for help from my employer and was told that as vacancies come available in the system, I may bid on them in competition and if successful move on then. Other than that, if I could get a psychologist or medical doctor to layout restrictions to my work then the employer will act to ensure that I don't get put in a position to do those things. They just don't understand it. The duty thing I have already dealt with, if I can't do it, I tell my boss and he has no problem with it.

So what is the issue you ask? How about using all your energies and time off for driving five hours one way up and down a highway? You should be using these energies to rebuild your immune system, take away any mental fatigue and just enjoy life to whatever degree possible. You may add that this highway is famous for fatalities and idiots behind the wheel. Forty times last year I spent running that road to get medical attention and therapy. Not sure how rested and revitalized you would be if you had to do that. Well the answer is, not at all!

After a battle with Cancer it takes years to build back a beaten body and the work doesn't end necessarily when you walk out the treatment room door. In many cases, your immune system has been compromised and your mind has been through countless traumas in the whole affair. In many cases the work begins when you walk out the treatment room door. Picture in your mind, an old dog at the SPCA that you can tell has been beaten and abused. Every time you bend to pet it, the dog cowers and cringes at the thought of another hit or kick in the ribs coming its way, which is all it knows. That is how I feel today, I hurt so deep inside it's hard to think I can heal and go on. I know I will though. Eventually it will happen. I have the love and support of a beautiful woman in my corner and I have three beautiful children to watch grow up and live out their dreams. If that isn't something to go on for, I don't know what is.

Sometimes however, you need another helping hand along the way to pull you up that last little bit of the mountain. You have been loyal, dedicated, and maybe even at times and in my case to the detriment of my family life put everything into the job. You hope for compassion, understanding, and good will, but you find it isn't there. You are just a number with another number out there available to replace you when you are gone. Your years of service and loyalty don't mean anything except with the people you have worked side by side with. You still have a lot to offer your profession and in many ways you are a leader in the field blazing new trails. But you will take work to support, and it seems have become high maintenance to your employer so you are told you cannot receive any special considerations unless it is specifically directed by a medical professional. It doesn't matter how much sense it makes, in the land of policy and bureaucracy present in all aspects of our everyday lives, that is just the way things are. Deal with it.

This exact scenario may not occur in your situation, but it is a real situation and you may encounter a similar challenge. Although people can be sympathetic to your cause, policy and bureaucracy may tie their hands and leave you to fend for yourself as I feel I am. You will hear things like use this time to reflect and assess your life. I didn't expect to be handed the key to the city, I just hoped for some ideas or options on how to find a mutually beneficial solution to the situation with my employer. I did not hear things such as, have you thought about this type of position or tell me what you excel at and maybe we can work together to find something that benefits both us and you. Having a job you love is fantastic and envious of all around you. Having a job you love that you cannot do anymore is sad. I am disappointed with the outcome of it all but mature enough to reflect, assess and determine what is best for me. The bottom line is there is no job in the world worth killing yourself over so figure out what is best for you and approach life in a different manner if need be.

Chapter 45

You Will Never Be the Same

Prepare for life changes, Cancer is a life changer in all areas of your life. Nothing will be the same again. I have struggled for days as to what to leave you with as a final sort of message so let me just say this. It isn't contagious, really it isn't, and it touches everyone at one time or another. We need to be able to talk about it freely and figure out how to make it better for all those that it does impact today, because tomorrow is too late.

Contact the Author

I would enjoy hearing from you, if you would like to send me a note or drop me a line I can be reached at My3Bellybuttons@hotmail.ca

Thanks for reading,

John Bruce

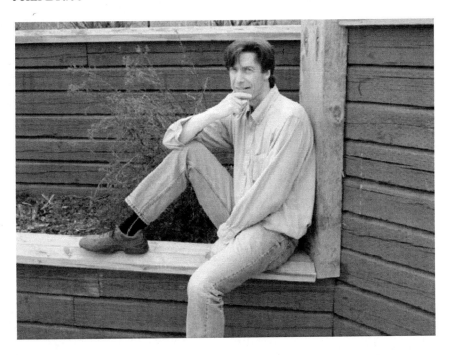